What's Cooking Within?

A SPIRITUAL COOKBOOK

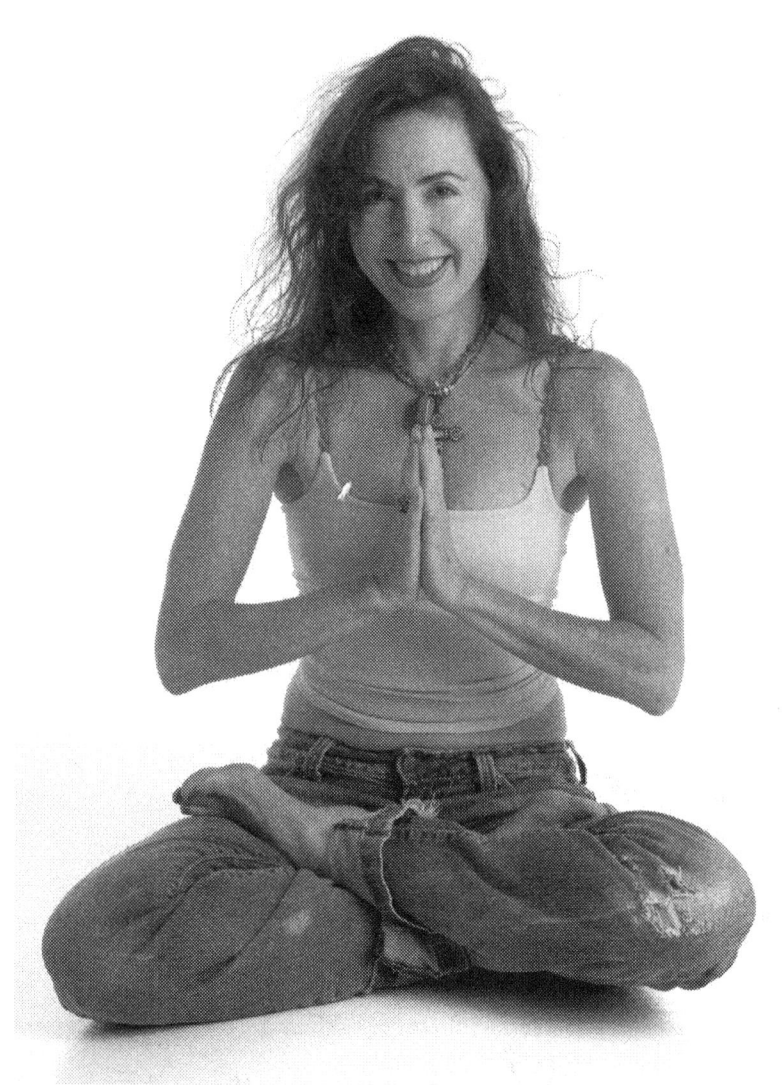

Published by Virtual Bookworm
www.virtualbookworm.com

Copyright © 2004 by Jyl Auxter
All rights reserved.

Photographs: Copyright © JohnDurant.com

Design by Jennifer Bacon
Cover by Niki Bradley

ISBN: 1-58939-481-x

Manufactured in the United States

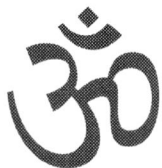

*D*ear Kindred Spirits:

It is an honor to share this spiritual cookbook with you. It is a book that I hope will provide you support and sustenance on your spiritual journey. Why have I chosen to combine a cookbook with spiritual guidance and yoga? Because as we embrace yoga, meditation and prayer, our human vibration, awareness and consciousness will shift toward a higher spiritual self. As we change, we leave behind our old, worn out, false selves. Many things will change including our eating habits, the people we want to be around and the things in our life that bring us joy. We may find that the food and drink that we used to crave no longer satisfies us. The focus of our awareness will be on making choices that are to our highest and best good, and this will include the foods we choose to consume. My goal with this book is to facilitate this transition to allow our rebirth to occur. My hope for us all is to allow a future of healthiness, holiness and happiness.

Love and Namaste,

This book is dedicated to my mother, who died April 8th, 2003, and also to my beloved father, who could not bear to live without his soul mate, and died January 11, 2004. Married sixty-one years, I have never met two people more in love than Bob and Vanda Auxter. I am forever grateful to my first and best teachers.

ACKNOWLEDGMENTS

*T*hank You to…

- ♥ *All the souls* who had the courage to walk through the door of 914 Highland Avenue, Del Mar, CA. Without you, Yoga by Jyl might never have happened!

- ♥ *Rick Jelusich* for intuitively coaching me to consider writing this cookbook.

- ♥ *Gina, Karen, Margo, Julie, Kathi, Gigi and others* who greatly encouraged me and gently prodded me by constantly asking, "Where are those recipes?"

- ♥ *Dolores,* you are my most loyal and disciplined student, and it certainly shows. Your help in editing and your final readings were certainly invaluable.

- ♥ *Cat,* your gentle soul and creative eye really supported me in my writing.

- ♥ *John,* you always make me feel beautiful in front of the camera.

- ♥ *Jen…* God surely sent you to help me. You put your life on hold to transform my writings into something worth reading. I will be forever grateful.

DISCLAIMER

"What's Cooking Within" is a guide written to help you follow and honor your truth. The ideas, suggestions and procedures herein are my truth. Go within, connect with your own voice, and consult a health care professional for matters regarding your health.

Neither the author nor the publisher will be liable for any loss or damage allegedly arising from information in this book.

CONTENTS

Starting Within...1

Yoga by Jyl...5

Embarking on the Journey 9

Components of Yoga 13

Meditation... 25

Chakras 29

Doshas...41

Yoga and Dinner 57

Begin Healing with Foods.. 65

Create Your New Life 75

Food to Feed the Soul 83

Entrees and Side Dishes..87

Salads 125

Soups 133

Breakfast 151

Breads 157

Desserts 163

Sauces & Salad Dressings 181

Eight Limbs of Ashtanga Yoga 201

Resources 205

Index.. 207

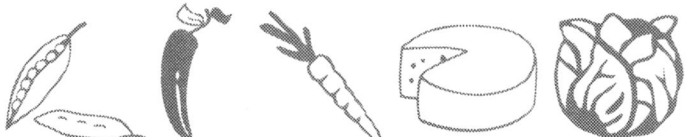

Part One

THE JOURNEY WITHIN

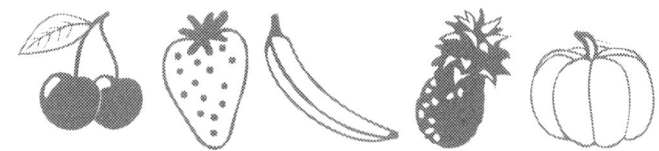

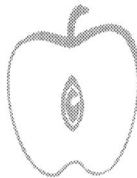

Starting Within

What lies behind us and what lies before us are tiny matters compared to what lies within us.

--Ralph Waldo Emerson

I realize now, looking back on my life, that I thought I was doing quite well. I had an undergraduate degree in nutrition, so I made it a point to eat healthfully. My work toward a graduate degree was in psychology, so I had completely analyzed my family of origin. I was an avid runner and marathoner, had a great corporate job and did yoga weekly. I thought I was healthy, because I had good eating habits and looked very fit, but over time, I found myself having a healing crisis at a young age. Sometimes you can be doing everything right and still get sick! I became so ill that I was forced to stop and review my life; to go within.

I took time out to heal. I scrutinized my diet, practiced more yoga, received healing energy and bodywork, got rid of my boyfriend and prayed a lot. On my path, I was fortunate enough to meet a number of spiritual teachers who counseled me and supported me in my own personal healing. Now I would like to share with you the lessons I've learned on my healing journey.

My healthier lifestyle emerged when I decided to become a yoga teacher. One night, I found myself in a yoga studio in a typical low-budget shopping center, lying in resting pose and thinking, "What would be the most enjoyable way to do yoga in the coolest environment?" I kept visualizing myself in beautiful intimate surroundings with a teacher giving me a foot and head massage. Following the practice, after the massage, I could just sit up and have someone serve me a gourmet meal by candlelight. That night, I went back home and thought, "I could create that!" Since having that epiphany, I have taught yoga classes in my home and served organic gourmet meals to hundreds of hungry students over the years.

> *Difficulties prepare you for victory. Disease prepares you for health. Confusion prepares you for clarity. Hopelessness prepares you for purpose. Failure prepares you for success. Poverty prepares you for prosperity. Criticism prepares you for acceptance. Pain prepares you for joy. Anger prepares you for forgiveness. Ignorance prepares you for truth. Loneliness prepares you for love. Love prepares you to stand face to face with God. God is the one who sends whatever it is you need to be prepared.*
>
> *It is called HEALING.*
>
> *[Only God and YOU heal YOU.]*
>
> *The Big Book of Faith* by Iyanla Vanzant

When I started my new business, "Yoga by Jyl", and my life started shifting, I wanted to share some of my experiences and changes with others. My passion is to help my students get in touch with their truth and their lives through yoga. I've found that this experience will lead them to want to put the right foods into their bodies. My students always tell me "BUT I do eat right!" What does "eating right" really mean? I have seen so many students change their lives by knowing their truth. Before we start cooking, I would like to share my life and some of my truths.

How did you start your journey within?

How have you incorporated healing into your life?

Notes from Within: _____

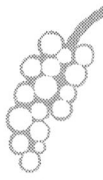

Yoga by Jyl

Be in this world but not of it... go within to discover the true you. Then let the world see it!

--Jesus (& Jyl!)

LIFE BY JYL

I was born in the Midwest and raised on a small vegetable farm in a town of five hundred people. My father, like his father before him, was a farmer. I watched my mother pick her own vegetables, can them and make delicious homemade juices and sauces. I grew up knowing what kind of meat was going into my body, because I saw what our cattle were fed. Each morning I would go to the chicken coop and bring in freshly laid eggs for our breakfast.

When I grew up and became a young woman, life on the farm finally came to an end and out of the nest I flew. After college, I sought success - as many of us do - in the business realm. For about fifteen years, I was in my corporate suit with briefcase in hand. When it was time for my soul to change direction and do my life's work, it was quite an interesting transition.

I remember writing the word courage on my bathroom wall and thinking that it must be courage that I lacked, because I was still stuck in the same old corporate madness. I was just about to see how much courage I really had. I prayed to God one evening, asking to be shown my new life path. With all my heart and soul, I was ready for a change. That is when life got very interesting and a bit tricky. Soon, as you will discover, I found myself knee-deep in my own drama, a drama that seemed like it would never end.

Seeking spiritual guidance, I turned to a popular book from a well-known local author and spiritual guru. I decided to do some workshops with this famous guru and soon was offered a job at his new center as the marketing director. I was thrilled and was sure that I had received the job for which I had been praying. But I quickly learned that even in a spiritual organization people are still human. After several negative experiences, I chose to leave.

A year after my experience, I was approached by a law firm that asked me to come forward to help another woman, who claimed she had been mistreated by the center and this guru. I shared my own experiences with them, and before I knew it, I was involved in litigation. This experience destroyed my trust in spiritual teachers, gurus and their organizations. Maybe I should say I promptly took them down off the pedestals on which I had placed them.

On the last day of the trial, my lawyer wrote the word courage on the blackboard in front of the jury. I took one look at that word and broke out in tears in the courtroom. The first statement out of his mouth was that his client had shown a lot of courage to come forward with the truth. As difficult as this situation was, I learned some very positive lessons from it. I learned that I truly had a lot of courage. I had stood up both for myself and for someone else. I also learned that nothing in life is good or bad. It just is what it is: an experience. And perhaps most importantly, I learned how important it is to go within, to find, and then live, your own truth.

But God hadn't stopped getting my attention. In addition to the trial, my best girl friend was killed in a violent auto accident. My boyfriend was misbehaving and causing me heartache once again. My corporate high tech job was literally killing me, and the idea of getting up in the morning to report to work was becoming more and more difficult. Finally, to top it all off, I had a golf ball size lump on the left side of my neck, which my doctor thought might be cancerous. But, amidst all this trauma, I would soon find out that this would truly be the beginning of my new life. I was awakening and embarking on a very special journey. This was my wake up call. Many people get their own wake up calls, but neglect to pick up the phone!

STARTING OVER

Fortunately, I did heed my wake up call, and it led me to great emotional, mental and spiritual healing through yoga, bodywork, meditation and eating differently. An outgrowth of my healing was that I decided to take a risk and create my yoga business, Yoga by Jyl.

Stepping out on my own proved to be less threatening than I thought it would be. By aligning myself with my higher truth, I found myself experiencing amazing coincidences. It seemed incredibly easy to let it unfold. I soon found myself on Lifetime TV, with a growing client base and a thriving business. Stepping into the fear brought me to a place of greater truth and faith.

As a yoga teacher, I strongly emphasize the spiritual, emotional and physical aspects of life while students are on the yoga mat. Just in case my students are experiencing a wake up call themselves, I remind them, "Yoga begins the minute class is over and you walk back into the world. Can you surrender into a calm place within, while there is craziness all around you?"

It is exciting for me to see how yoga has become so popular. While many people want to be yoga teachers these days, few realize that the minute you become the teacher, you become the student. It is one of the hardest jobs I have ever had. I always say, "You can't wipe the tear of another unless you yourself have wept." Or better yet… "You can't be the AA counselor if you have never been a drunk"… you get the picture! I get to be the teacher and healer, because I am doing the healing.

Healing through yoga can be serious business, so I decided to create a soothing and serene environment with candlelight, lavender-filled silk eye pillows, hand-knit blankets made by my talented mother and a healthy gourmet dinner to soften the experience. I nurture and feed my students with the blessings in the kitchen and God's energy that flows through me. An evening yoga session with Jyl goes something like this: soft candlelight, a guided meditation with a spiritual reading, a powerful asana practice and a mindful seated meditation followed by a healing foot and head massage with essential oils. All this is capped off with a healthy, organic gourmet dinner, a more indulgent dessert and a glass of wine. Sometimes we do our yoga practice to live music by my friend Barton. There is nothing like doing yoga to live heartfelt music, especially when the musician is Barton!

What wake-up calls have you experienced? How have you listened?

Where do you find courage in your life?

Notes from Within: _____

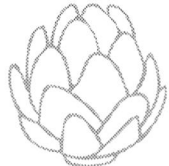

Embarking on the Journey

Before starting the yoga journey, all students must take a private yoga session with the teacher!!

When I first began teaching, I didn't insist on having everyone take a private session. Then, one night, I learned a huge lesson. The room was packed, and we were well into the practice, when I noticed one of the students was struggling. Little did I know, she was about to go into a diabetic seizure.

When she collapsed on the floor, her friends, who knew she was diabetic, ran to get her medication. We were able to revive her, but the experience was extremely disconcerting. Not having the medical information on this student put me in the position of not knowing how to respond to this dangerous situation. Had I known about her condition, I could have addressed it before the class even began.

Now, whenever I have a new student, I always get their medical background and have them sign a health waiver. I take the time to get to know them and their bodies. It is important to have compatibility and intimacy with my students, since we will not only be having a physical workout, but also an emotional, mental and spiritual workout as well. Taking the time to sit with my students adds real value to the practice. I highly recommend this to all yoga teachers.

When students come for their private session, they are all at different places in their journey. After going over their medical history and a written handout on the foundations of yoga, I take the time to customize each asana, or yoga posture. This not only addresses their physical limitations, but also gives them the confidence to follow the practice and listen to their bodies.

Looking back at the private sessions, they have all been unique. Sometimes students needed a healing session before we even discussed yoga. Some had to be fed emotionally, spiritually and physically. I literally remember making breakfast for one of my students before we could begin the private session. Some just needed to vent. All these private sessions were God-given opportunities to meet and support different souls on their paths.

PICKING A PERFECT YOGA TEACHER

Many new yoga students tell me they use a video to learn yoga. While there are some beautiful videos in the marketplace, I really encourage you to seek out a studio and a teacher when you are just getting started. Sit still, pray, go within and ask the universe to direct you to the perfect teacher. I once had a student tell me that he visited every yoga studio in the city before deciding to practice with me. He said that my style really felt good to him.

That is exactly what yoga is about; your job is to know what makes you feel good. I used to go to a yoga studio where I didn't enjoy the environment or the strong egos in the room. Now as I think about it, I didn't even enjoy the teacher. This doesn't create a great yoga experience and certainly won't keep anyone coming back for more.

When you are looking for your perfect yoga teacher, there are a few things to keep in mind. Find someone who you will be compatible with, who will help you grow emotionally, mentally and spiritually. Yoga will take you on a journey, and you want someone who will help guide you through the rough spots. It's also great to have someone to remind you of how far you've come and to celebrate your successes.

You want your teacher to be someone who will coach you, help you to honor your body and keep you safe on the sticky mat. This will keep you coming back. A good teacher can help you get the most out of the yoga postures. A good teacher will offer you a foundation in yoga and teach you to have faith in the process.

I always discuss faith during my students' first private yoga session. A person must have faith in the practice of yoga and in life. You must believe, at some level, that the universe is really on your side. Blind faith is helpful for beginning yoga students. It really can take years to see any results from all the hard work. While I have been studying yoga for over twenty years, I still sometimes question the true benefits of the practice, but I keep coming back, knowing how good yoga makes me feel.

It can be hard to keep faith in life during painful times. Yoga realigns the body, and as it is healing, this realignment can be painful. I truly believe that pain does purify us on many levels. Faith develops over time as you begin to discover that the universe does have your best interests at heart, and one way or another, life always works out!

A very type A woman came to me for some private yoga sessions. After about three months, she wanted to know why she wasn't further along in the practice. This was a woman who was searching for quick fixes, but yoga is a life-long process that opens the heart and heals the body. This life-hardened woman simply needed love to break down the walls around her so the healing could begin. Sometimes in life, just allowing people to see your own faith in the unknown is the best and only gift you can give.

> *Belief is the food of the believer; it is the sustenance of his faith. It is on belief he lives, not on food and water. Faith is the ABC of the realization of God; this faith begins by prayer.*
>
> --Hazrat Inayat Khan

Yoga is multi-faceted and will change your life. I always tell my students, as they begin their journey, don't start yoga unless you are ready for some major changes. Can you allow change in your life? I realize that change can be very scary for all of us, and most of us do not embrace change. I have seen some of my clients change jobs, start their own companies, heal their bodies and leave worn-out unhealthy relationships. In my own life, I have left corporate America, started my own company and healed my overly stressed body. I have experienced one of the greatest challenges in life, the death of both my parents. My father would always say to me, "Williper (my nickname), we all have to pay taxes and die someday, so learn to go with the flow that life brings."

Allowing those life changes to occur can be challenging. Learning how to stay in the flow of life, without denying that hard-earned change or shift, can certainly bring up some emotions. During private sessions, I offer tools that help students embrace those changes. I not only teach my students about yoga, but also other related subjects like meditation and prayer, chakras and doshas. These are all tools that help my students learn more about their truth and speed them on their life's journey through their ever-changing existence.

What tools are in your life supporting you on your journey?

Notes from Within: _____

What does faith mean to you?

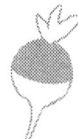

Components of Yoga

Ashtanga Yoga is 99% practice, 1% theory.

--Pattabhi Jois

YOGA HISTORY

Yoga has been around for about 5,000 years. It all started with a race of Sanskrit (the sacred language of India) speaking people called the Aryans. The Aryans inhabited the Indus Valley and developed a new science; the science of the mind. They were the first people to use a systematic mode of inquiry to study their own nature and purpose. From the Aryans and their discoveries came yoga.

Some 2,500 years later, a sage named Patanjali created the sutras, written descriptions of yoga that survived the Aryan culture. There are a total of 195 sutras and these writings address the nature of the body, the nature of thoughts, the nature of consciousness, the nature of the breath and the supernatural powers. So, in addition to the physical discipline and workout that we know yoga to be, yoga is also based on a science of the mind and much more.

Once a student has mastered the basic asanas (postures), there is so much more to learn and practice. I have a student who is always telling me that he needs to take on more yoga. What he means is he needs to advance the asana practice. That is fine, but if he really wanted to embrace yoga, he might consider embracing the sutras. Yoga is not just about performing the right postures. It's about going within and embracing your truth and your life, through the asanas.

YOGA IS THE PERFECT WORKOUT

In my lifetime, I have tried just about every sport. I like to say that I am a recovered marathon runner. Running served as my main physical outlet for many years, until I discovered yoga. I found yoga to be the most complete workout, because it provided a window into my inner self and added more balance than I had ever experienced in my entire life. I have tried many styles of Hatha yoga. For many years, I practiced the more structured Iyengar yoga and obtained my teacher training and knowledge through this practice. Kundalini yoga helped me to see the power of a healing practice. Ashtanga yoga, the form of yoga I currently teach, is probably the closest to my heart, because it is a very intense workout, in every sense of the word. It has taken the place of my marathon running and changed my life forever. To this day, I believe it is yoga - more than any other thing - that has kept me healthy and balanced.

All forms of yoga are worth trying. In the years I have been practicing yoga, I have discovered that the key is to find a practice that suits your body type. Now that yoga has become so popular, it's important not to lose sight of the true purpose of yoga. Remember to use yoga as a method to truly discover yourself, as the Aryan people intended. Be your own teacher.

Not long ago, a highly regarded Brahman guru from India came to San Diego. In India, a Brahman is thought to be a person who possesses great spiritual powers. I had been waiting for years to meet and practice with him. The students I knew who went off to India to study with this guru always seemed to come back with more insight and a better yoga practice. I never knew if it was the experience of India or the yoga that created the transformation. When I finally got to meet this supreme Brahman, my experience proved to be quite different from what I had expected.

Three days before the guru's visit, I was awakened in the early morning hours by a loud voice in my head. The voice kept saying, "Don't look for the guru; find the guru within." Of course I thought I was going crazy, but after doing the practice with this supreme Brahman, I came to realize that we are all supreme beings. I encourage my students to listen to their inner voices and to let the yoga be their teacher or guru. My truth in this lifetime is about going inside myself to discover God and the teacher.

Who are you I say... find out and do yoga.

So while a good yoga teacher is important, it's essential to have someone who is in line with your higher spiritual, emotional, physical and mental self, a teacher who can help you uncover the real guru... YOU!

Buddha's last words were recorded as... "Be a lamp unto yourself." He didn't say go running to this teacher or that center... he said, "Be a lamp unto yourself." Yes, just for the record, Buddha had many teachers along the way. I guess that is why he left behind this important message on his dying day. It will never be about what the great masters have to say about you. The responsibility is yours. What will you say about you? Make sure to turn on your own lamp, and let it shine.

The word Yoga means Union... Union between you and your beautiful higher realm.

BENEFITS OF A COMMITTED YOGA PRACTICE

　　Lowers your blood pressure

　　Calms your nerves

　　Offers a sense of peace in your life

　　Heals the body

　　Balances the body

　　Great workout for strength and flexibility

　　Changes your diet

　　Helps you lose weight

　　Helps burn toxins out of the body

　　Creates a spiritual awakening

　　Creates a healthy lifestyle

　　Preamble to meditation

　　Creates changes in your life that are for your highest good

　　Makes you feel so wonderful

　　Introduces you to your higher self and your life's purpose

BEFORE YOU START YOUR YOGA PRACTICE - LEARN THE BASICS.

BASIC COMPONENTS OF YOGA

　　Breath

　　Edge

　　Prana & Bandhas

　　Drishti

　　Asanas

　　Yoga Therapy

BREATH

　　A good teacher will continually remind you that the breath is the practice of yoga. Yoga means union between you and the breath (spirit). The method of breathing in the Ashtanga practice is called Ujjayi breathing, or victorious breath. This method of breathing requires that you breathe through your nose and allow your inhale to whirl in back of the throat. Inhale a long deep breath. It opens the heart and flows down to the base of the spine. Follow inhales by deep exhales. Squeeze the air out of the root of the spine. Inhales and exhales should be effortless. You will be able to hear the hissing sound of your breath throughout the practice.

The goal of the breath is to have inhales and exhales become equal in depth and length. Inhales represent receiving. Are you a person who can receive the gifts that life offers? Exhales represent giving. Can you give without expecting anything in return? This is surely an easy concept, but is very hard to apply in life. So the goal is to receive and give equally in life, creating a breath that flows and awakens the body.

> The Breath warms up the body and prepares you for the practice of yoga.
>
> The Breath cleanses and purifies the body.
>
> The Breath keeps the body safe while performing the asanas or yoga postures.
>
> The Breath clears the mind of thoughts. Negative thoughts can be harmful to your health.
>
> The Breath connects you to a higher force... God, Spirit, Jesus, Buddha or whatever you believe is your higher source.

As you start the breathing, be patient. This might be one of the biggest challenges in yoga. Blowing your nose before the practice is helpful. An essential oil that I have found works well if you are congested is Eucalyptus oil. Place 2-3 drops in your hands or on a tissue. Rub your hands together, stick your nose in your hands or place the tissue under your nose and inhale deeply. True essential oils can be very powerful. If your skin is sensitive, make sure to wash your hands afterwards.

THE EDGE

After the breath, the edge is surely the most important component of yoga. I always like to spend time with my new students discussing the edge. While in the yoga postures, go to your edge. On a scale of one to ten, with ten being "I'm hurting myself," find the edge in your body at seven. This should be the point where it hurts "so good."

I often refer to the edge as Pandora's Box. In other words, every trauma in your life is hidden neatly at your edge. It has often been said that we hold all of our emotions in our body. C. Norman Shealy, M.D., Ph.D., is a neurosurgeon who discovered, in his work with patients in chronic pain, that at the root of most illness is an unresolved emotion. This pain is known as your edge.

Yoga is such a powerful tool in helping you discover your repressed emotions that it can actually free your body from them. I ask my students to go to the tension or pain in their bodies, to breathe and release, then find a new edge. I have noticed that if I haven't had a discussion with new students about the edge, they get frustrated with yoga and don't have the courage to continue the practice. They may even hurt themselves if they approach their edge too aggressively or forget to breathe. One must have courage to go into the pain and discover the real emotional edge that's behind it.

One edge always leads to another. The question is not if you are ready to deal with the physical pain of yoga postures, but are you truly ready to deal with your true self and your life's issues… THE REAL PAIN! Sometimes, when you find an emotional or physical edge, it doesn't feel so good, like pressing on a bruise. What is the point? You may feel as though you are only producing more pain. But, by embracing your edges, it aids the body in eliminating harmful emotions that can lead to stagnation and illness. Once you have released the emotion living at your edge, you will have created a whole new body that has room for peace, harmony, joy and growth.

> Spiritual Edge… having faith EVEN when the money runs out!
>
> Physical Edge… ouch!
>
> Mental Edge… keeping all thoughts pure and peaceful.
>
> Emotional Edge… DEAL with your greatest fear either now or later.

When you are experiencing the edge during your yoga practice, watch for helpful teachers. While I have been in many yoga postures in my lifetime and have had some helpful adjustments, I have also had many injuries as a result of them. In fact, the last adjustment I had, made by a well-meaning yoga teacher, left me on crutches. It blew out my knee joint, which required knee surgery! While it was very sobering to be hobbling around trying to teach yoga on crutches, the most disheartening thing was that my teacher at the time didn't believe his adjustment had caused my injury. Now I had really met my edge. As I spent five months recovering, I dealt with issues such as integrity, fear and frustration. When a very physical person, such as me, is forced to sit still for an extended amount of time it can be very trying on the nerves. I guess you might say I was grounded, and I learned a lot about myself in the process. I had opened my own Pandora's Box and all those lovely, unresolved life issues. The lesson to be learned from this is when you are at your edge, and your teacher wants to push you a little further, just say NO…. Please learn to practice healthy boundaries while you are in class, and if a teacher has a problem respecting those boundaries, then you may have the wrong teacher.

As you progress in your yoga practice, you will learn to release old emotions and let yourself go to a calmer inner place. Learn to allow yourself to experience true peace. Think of yoga as a form of therapy. Learn to be the observer. Observe yourself letting go of your worry, fear and anger. Worry, fear and anger are not welcomed in a body that does yoga.

Make sure to allow yourself to cry once in awhile during resting pose, the last posture of the yoga class. This is a sign that you are on your way to freedom. Recently, I had one of my students approach me after everyone had left class. She wanted to share that she was close to tears but felt uncomfortable crying. I reassured her that crying was part of the healing process. By bringing up emotions, yoga allows us to clear our bodies of past traumas.

PRANA & BANDHAS

Prana is life-force energy, or spiritual energy. The prana flows up through the spine creating a lighter brighter you. Prana is created in the base of the spine. By lifting the pelvis floor during the inhale, a yoga student begins to access this spiritual energy.

The way we move prana is through the bandhas. Bandhas, or locks, are engaged during the practice of yoga to direct the flow of this spiritual energy upwards. They help to keep you safe within the postures. Think of your spine as a tube of toothpaste. Apply pressure to the tube, and you move the paste. The same thing happens when you apply bandhas to your yoga practice. Life-force energy is moved. Healing energy has been released.

There are three bandhas, Mula Bandha, Uddiyana Bandha and Jalandhara Bandha. Mula Bandha is at the root of the spine. By lifting the pelvic floor, heat begins to warm the body. Uddiyana Bandha moves prana in the body and is located in the belly. By contracting the lower abdomen and pulling it inward and upward toward the spine, an internal cleansing and a blessing occur. Jalandhara Bandha is located at the throat. The throat area of the body holds a lot of emotions. By placing pressure on this area, we concentrate the prana. When the pressure is released, the energy can flow freely up through the body. Balance and mental clarity can be obtained by releasing this lock.

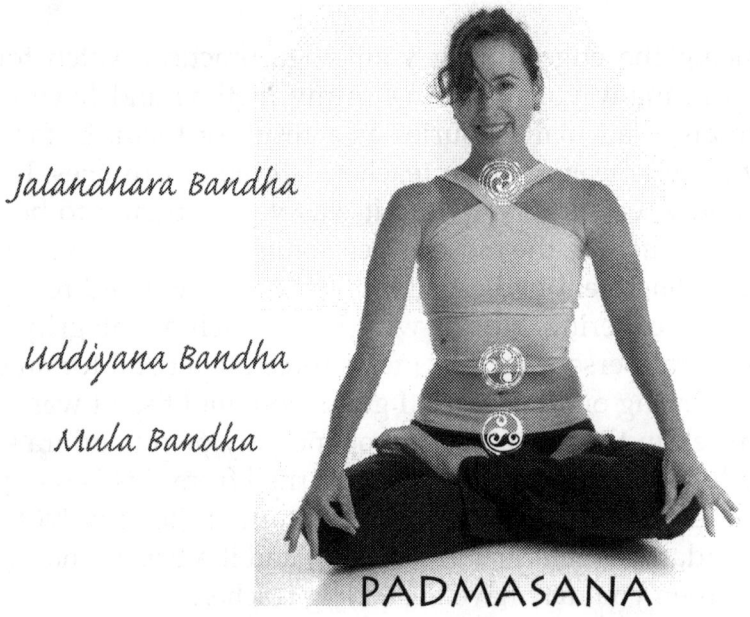

PADMASANA

The Hindus of India believe that there is a metaphorical lotus flower at the base of your spine, and in the middle of the flower sleeps a powerful serpent. When a yogi begins the breath and engages the bandhas, the serpent starts to awaken and rises up the spine, creating a more enlightened yogi. In the yoga world, this is referred to as "Kundalini rising."

Like the practice of Ujjayi breathing, bandhas take time to develop. You have to feel the movement of prana in your own body. Every yoga posture is designed to help you feel the bandhas. An ability to access the bandhas is essential to get into some of the more advanced postures. By being consistent in your yoga practice, you can develop a deeper understanding and sense for how the bandhas work. Until they become natural in your practice, each time you start a new yoga class set your intention to be mindful of the bandhas, and watch what happens! Richard Freeman, a highly respected ashtanga yoga teacher, once said, "Yoga begins first in the mind, then on the sticky mat."

DRISHTI

"You've got to know where you are going in life in order to get there." When was the last time you sat with yourself and imagined your future? This message applies in life and to yoga. Drishti is the Sanskrit word for gaze or focus. By directing your attention and gaze to a certain area, the movement will flow toward that area. The drishti prepares the muscles for movement. Let's say you are going to look up at your hand, the upward gaze prepares the muscles in the neck. Each posture in yoga has a specific drishti, and when in doubt simply look at the nose! The nose always knows…

ASANAS

The poses, or yoga postures, are called asanas. The asanas combine the breath and movement to develop strength and flexibility. Each posture, or asana, is performed slowly. When students are new, the asanas are not held very long, and the flow seems a bit faster. As your practice develops, so does your strength and flexibility. This enables you to flow slowly and effortlessly through each yoga posture. In this country, we place a great deal of importance on the poses, treating yoga like exercise. Please try not to fall into this line of thinking, because if you do, you will truly miss the beauty and the greatest benefits of the practice.

Many people who are new to yoga question whether or not it is right for them, because they are not flexible. My response is always, "Can you breathe?" Yoga is about breathing, and it doesn't really matter if you are flexible or not. When I first started yoga, I could barely bend forward and touch my knees. After more than a dozen marathons, I found my body locked up and distressed. I had actually run my body into the ground. With consistent practice, I soon discovered my flexibility.

Not only did I have physical limitations from all the marathons I had run, but I encountered a few emotional and mental limitations as well. The healthier I became, and the more yoga I did, I found a certain softness that replaced the shield around my heart, the fear around my hips and the lack of confidence in my shoulders.

YOGA POSTURES:

Standing (vitality postures)

Sitting (calming postures)

Inversions/Upside down (nervous system postures)

Restorative (restful postures)

Back bends (heart opening postures)

Twisting (cleansing postures)

Balance (lightness postures)

A new friend, and fellow yoga teacher, once reminded me that the shoulder stand is the queen of asanas, and the headstand is the king of asanas. These are very powerful postures and are very beneficial to the body. If you are a beginner, take your time and always ask for your teacher's guidance, so you can safely begin to feel the posture. Both of these powerful asanas are done at the end of the practice. Think of them as postures of completion. Remember to allow yourself to become the king or queen in your own life.

YOGA THERAPY

Yoga therapy, sometimes referred to as Yoga Chikitsa, is putting all the above yoga components together to create a happier, healthier, wiser and whole you. Yoga therapy combines psychology and the ancient healing practice of yoga. Every time you do yoga, a new healthier form of you is created. You become a more balanced person. Try to keep the ego out of your yoga practice. Try to keep the critical voices to a soft roar. Allow your edges to guide you through your own therapy session while on your sticky mat.

I had a student who was always fussing with herself during class. When we were able to do a private session together, I discovered that her mind was so filled with harsh, overly critical voices that she was unable to find pleasure in yoga. I asked her to breathe into this craziness, and the more she breathed and honored where she was, the more peace would follow during the practice. Soon after, this student returned and told me that she was able to use the breathing techniques with great success. Use yoga to heal the body, the mind and open your heart to a kinder, more peaceful internal voice. You will not only discover a new voice within, but a much more balanced body.

Traditional psychotherapy is being replaced not only by the practice of yoga, but also by a new body-mind approach to emotional well being known as somatic psychology. This type of therapy centers on wellness using the breath, body sensations and physical energy. Long hours spent talking about family abuse, shame, guilt and anger are now being replaced with a strong positive body-mind approach. The emphasis now is creating a positive internal dialogue, healthy skills, personal mastery and lasting happiness.

Happiness involves skills for everyday living that few people consistently practice. Instead of taking pride in our accomplishments, we tend to be self-critical. Instead of holding positive visions of the future, we run worst-case scenarios, thinking that's the way to be prepared for emergencies. Rather than regularly expressing appreciation to those we love, we find fault with them, hoping to make them "better".

The Pleasure Zone by Stella Resnick, Ph.D.

In addition to teaching yoga, I also offer spiritual energy healing. My work allows me to help my yoga students heal their edges. I call my work "Yoga Therapy by Jyl," of course! A therapy session with Jyl includes Reiki, Raindrop Therapy, Phoenix Rising and Theta Healing. When a student is going through a healing crisis, I am able to use one or more modalities to get to the core of their problems.

I can still remember a young energetic yoga student who came to me after class because her throat hurt. She mentioned that during the whole class, she felt like someone was strangling her. I suggested that a healing session might help her understand and overcome this feeling. The yoga therapy session proved to be very beneficial, and we were able to get to her core issue. My client was yearning to be heard, but was afraid to speak her truth, especially to her father. Yoga therapy forces you to take responsibility for your own health. Empowering yourself is truly the way to heal!

The following is a brief description of the components in a "Yoga Therapy by Jyl" healing session:

Yoga Therapy: *Yoga Therapy combines Phoenix Rising release work, Raindrop Oil Therapy, Theta Healing and Reiki. This is an intense but soothing healing session.*

Phoenix Rising Release Body Work: *Phoenix Rising involves passive yoga postures which help move energy and release emotions. Studies show that at the core of most disease there is an unresolved emotion. This work helps to free our bodies from unhealthy emotions. This bodywork brought back my own health during my healing crisis.*

Raindrop Oil Therapy: *This technique involves dripping healing essential oils directly onto the spine. The body is brought into balance, and its energy centers can be cleared and realigned. It will help reduce spinal inflammations and kill viruses that hibernate along the spinal column. It will also help to straighten any spinal curvature.*

Theta Healing: *This technique accesses a deep meditative brain state. A theta state is a very deep state of relaxation. This hypnotic state offers a person an opportunity to go within and obtain great levels of healing from their internal higher source.*

Reiki: *Reiki represents Universal Life Energy. When this energy is activated and applied for healing purposes, it accelerates the body's ability to heal ailments and opens the mind and spirit to the causes of diseases and pain.*

I will never underestimate the power of Reiki. One time I had a group of teenage soccer players come to do yoga. The first student in my studio was wearing a leg cast, so I placed my hands on her cast, while I instructed the others through the yoga practice. The next day, I got a call from the soccer coach asking me what I did to the girl with the cast. Oh boy, I thought, I'm in trouble now! The coach informed me that the girl went back to the doctor to have the cast checked, and to the surprise of the doctor, the leg didn't need the cast. When the doctor asked the girl what happened to her leg, she proudly announced that her yoga teacher had touched her leg and healed her. Later, my cute new student told me, "You should have seen the doctor's face when I told him you simply placed your hands on my leg." The miracles around Reiki are many!

YOGA STIR FRY RECIPE

Before preparing this dish, step into a warm shower or bath to relax the muscles. Make sure your nose is clear, and no food has been consumed for at least 3 hours.

Then begin with:

> *Smooth deep (Ujjayi) breathing*
> *Add a deep emotional edge*
> *Stir up three strong bandhas*
> *Chop and direct drishti*
> *Add a sprinkle of asanas*
> *Toss with love*

Serve on a large yoga mat

This dish, if consumed at least three times a week, will heal your body and add a youthful bliss to your life.

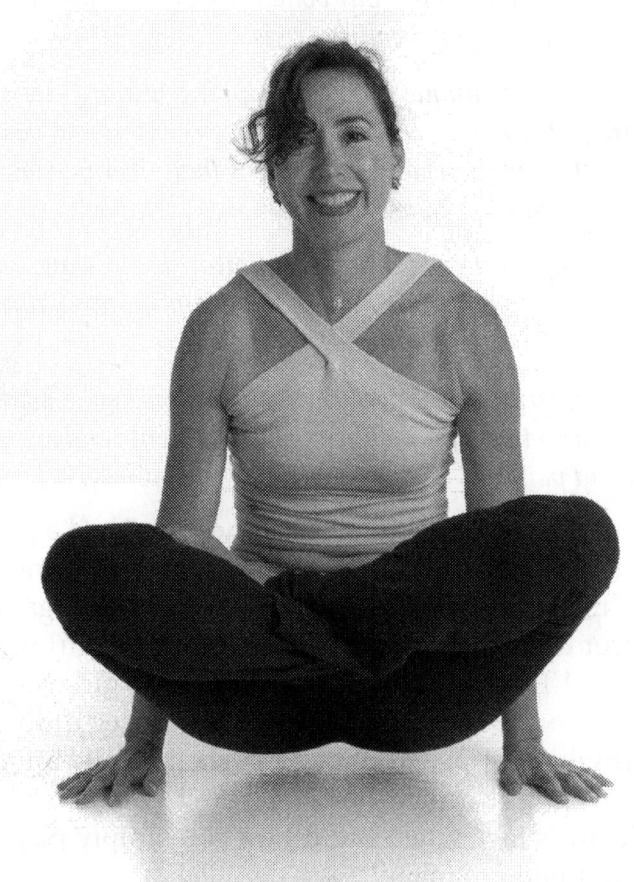

TOLASANA

What has your journey taught you about yourself?

Notes from Within: _____

Where is your drishti?

What are your edges in life? (physical, spiritual, mental & emotional)

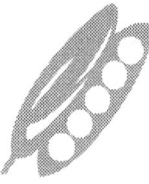

Meditation

Yoga teaches you Patience and Surrender.

Meditation is an integral part of yoga. This quiet time allows us to let go of our thoughts and quiet our minds. I am always surprised to hear my students say they are too busy to meditate; everyone can learn to meditate. Yoga is the preamble to sitting in meditation; meditation is the gift of yoga. Creating time in your day to meditate is a very loving and self-affirming act.

I truly think we have it completely backwards in our world. Our world teaches us to do. Do get up in the morning, do plug into the negative noise of television news, and do fill your life with so many tasks that by the end of the day you feel worthy because you are so stressed and exhausted. Dumb!

Did you ever notice that some people work so hard, never seem to get ahead and are always upset? Then there are others who seem so calm and are able to manifest everything they need. Many of those folks have learned to sit and meditate on their worldly desires. To them, the doing is creating the desired life in their thoughts. They are pre-paving the way to their desires by creating first in their minds.

What does this have to do with meditation, you may be asking, isn't meditation not thinking? Meditation is quieting the mental noise so that you can connect with your truth and God. Envision the mental chatter encased in a shimmering pearl-like cloud. As you sit with yourself, see your beautiful clouds passing by. Then you will start to hear thoughts. These thoughts are your truth, and as you connect with your essence and God, understanding your greater truth will be revealed.

As you become aware of this higher truth, you can start to DO life. By starting your day with meditation, you will allow life to unfold into the beauty that God intended. The doing will then become the receiving of gifts. Eventually, you will manifest these gifts of life during meditation. Meditation is communing with God or your life force - why would you want to miss out on this opportunity? Every answer to every question you have will be received when you meditate. Meditation is free for all of us, and it will change your life. Learning to meditate is one of the most challenging, yet simple, disciplines to develop. If you are really seeking your truth and a life of joy, learn to meditate.

My students with children laugh when I ask them to meditate. But learning to meditate can be one of the greatest gifts you can offer your children. One of my students, who came to me to learn to meditate, was from India. She told me the story of her parents, and how every morning they would make time to meditate. She and her siblings would honor that time and would not interrupt their parents. She now realizes what a gift this daily meditation was for her parents and regrets she did not learn it from them. So, parents, shift your thinking, and start being an example for your children.

BENEFITS OF MEDITATION

Great happiness

Great joy

Divine consciousness

Transformation

Healthy nervous system

Ability to focus

Ability to stay balanced

Physical healing

Creating a time to meditate is a great way to form a new habit and new life. Add meditation to your morning routine and be creative as you sit. Have a pen and paper available to write down anything significant that comes up in your thoughts. This allows you to reflect on your experience. Pour yourself a cup of coffee or tea. Make yourself very relaxed and comfortable - this should not be a time of torture!

I prefer to sit on a big furry pillow. I light some candles and have a mug of imported, jasmine green tea with creamy, vanilla soy milk and a spoonful of organic honey. I then settle in on my furry pillow, as if I were the Queen of Something, and sip my tea, connecting with my feelings and thoughts. I may spend some time just sitting before I am ready to write, do yoga, pray, meditate or pre-pave my day with positive thinking. Each day is different. I limit the morning meditation demands - no SHOULDS - and that keeps me coming back for more. After many months of this daily meditation, you will notice a complete change in your life. I use this simple exercise with many of my Yoga Therapy clients who are ready to take control of their own healing.

How can you bring meditation into your life?

Notes from Within: _____

Pre-pave your day in your mind. What does it look like?

Chakras

Yoga has been around for 5,000 years, healing bodies.

Yoga is a healing modality. The healing comes from moving and healing chakra energies. By having a good understanding of the chakras, it offers greater meaning to your yoga practice.

So what the heck is a chakra? Before that discussion, I have to tell you a funny story. When I first moved from North Carolina to Irvine, California, I was working in software, had received a promotion and life was pretty good - except for my love life. I was on the verge of breaking up with yet another boyfriend, when my friend Pete suggested I see a psychiatrist. No sooner had I walked into the doctor's office, when he looked at me like I had three heads and told me I had the energy of five people, I was psychic, I could see spirits and I would teach people about chakras.

I had only been in California for a couple of years, and for the first time since my move West I started to agree with what my family back on the farm had been saying; "There are a bunch of nut and berry eating crazies out there in California!" When my session was over, I wandered in a confused state toward my favorite gelato ice cream store. (Eating ice cream has always made me feel better!) I somehow managed to not tell anyone of my experience that day, and soon I would forget all about it.

Who would have guessed, years later, that I would no longer be in the software business, but I would be writing a spiritual cookbook and would be teaching my students about chakras. As I remember that day, that crazy doctor told me a great deal about my life, and all the details he shared with me have come true. My reason for telling you this story is to show you how important it is to stay open in life. Many of us have a hard time accepting that spirits talk through others, telling us about our lives. Learn not to discount anyone or anything you hear. Take these words of wisdom from someone who has seen the miracles inherent in each day.

Now back to the subject at hand: chakras. Along the spine there are seven main energy pockets, or emotional centers. When we begin our yoga practice, we begin fueling these emotional centers, or chakras, with life force energy, or prana. Yoga balances out the chakras. An illness is usually caused by unresolved emotional issues creating physical challenges around one of the chakras. It is our job to continue to go to our edge to discover the unresolved issues or emotions. Releasing the emotions and the negative thoughts at the edge heals the body.

Keep in mind that each asana, or yoga posture, has a chakra that it is designed to heal. In the following section, I have provided some yoga postures designed to help heal specific chakra energies. I have also described each chakra, given its Sanskrit name, listed the issues that correspond to that energy, the organs in the body that are affected and some physical dysfunctions caused by each unbalanced chakra. As you are reading about each chakra, think about how they relate to your life and health, then try each of the yoga postures, and have some fun healing.

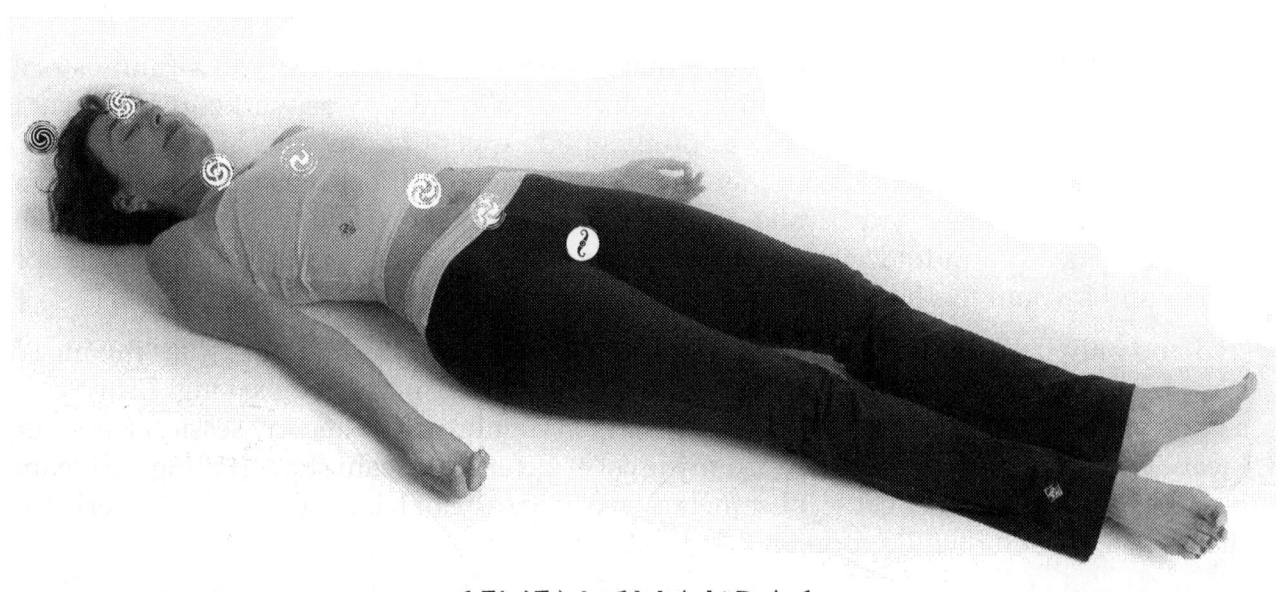

SEVEN CHAKRAS

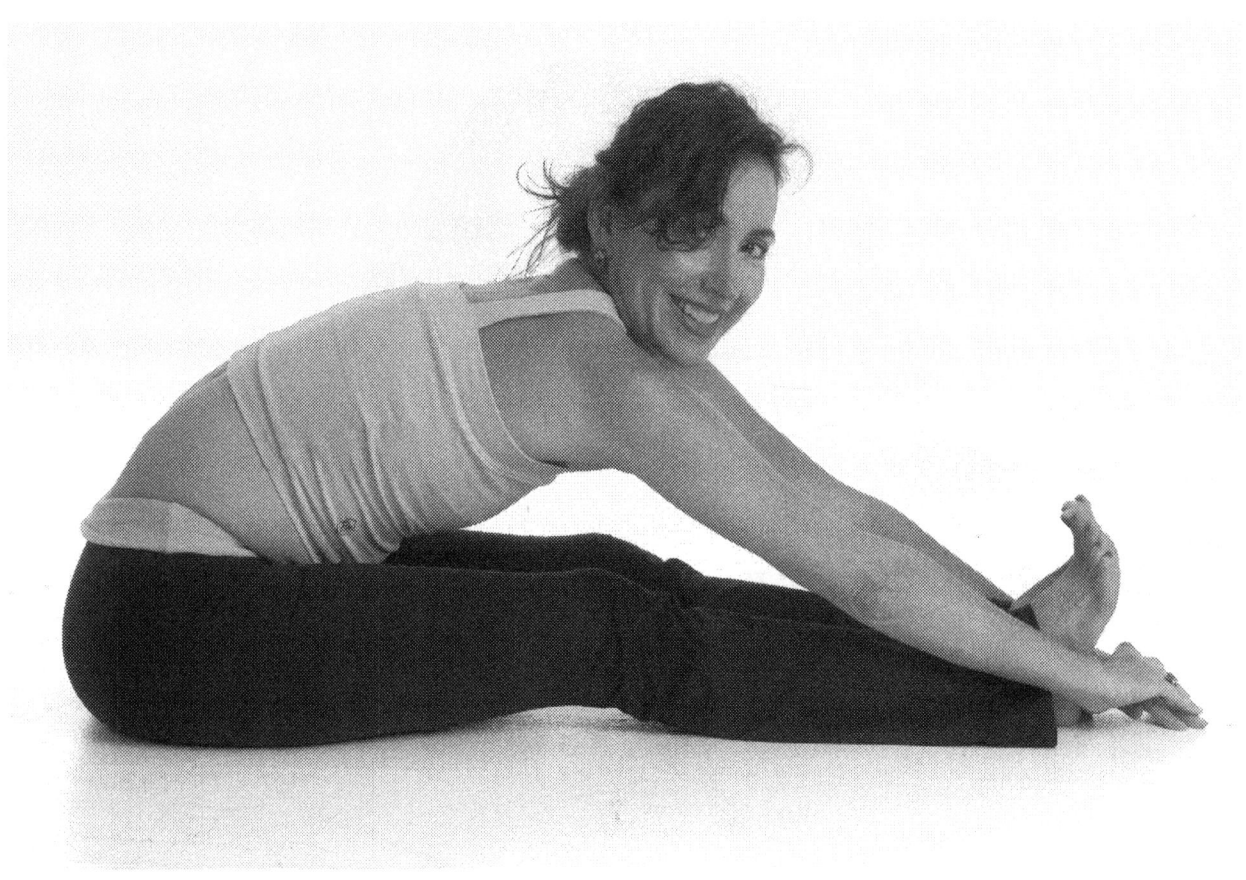

CHAKRA 1 MULADHARA

This chakra is found at the base of your spine, or at the root of your existence. The root chakra deals with family of origin issues. Did your family offer you support and security? Do you feel safe, and are you supported? Do you live a life of fear, or can you trust others? Do you feel helpless? Do you have the ability to cope?

Organ Systems Impacted: *spine, blood, immune system, bones*

Physical Dysfunctions: *sciatica, scoliosis, rectal problems, chronic fatigue, fibromyalgia, autoimmune disease, arthritis, skin problems*

Yoga Posture: *Sit on the floor with straight legs and tall, straight spine, inhale deeply to the base of your spine, exhale folding forward, bend your knees if the backs of your legs are tight.*

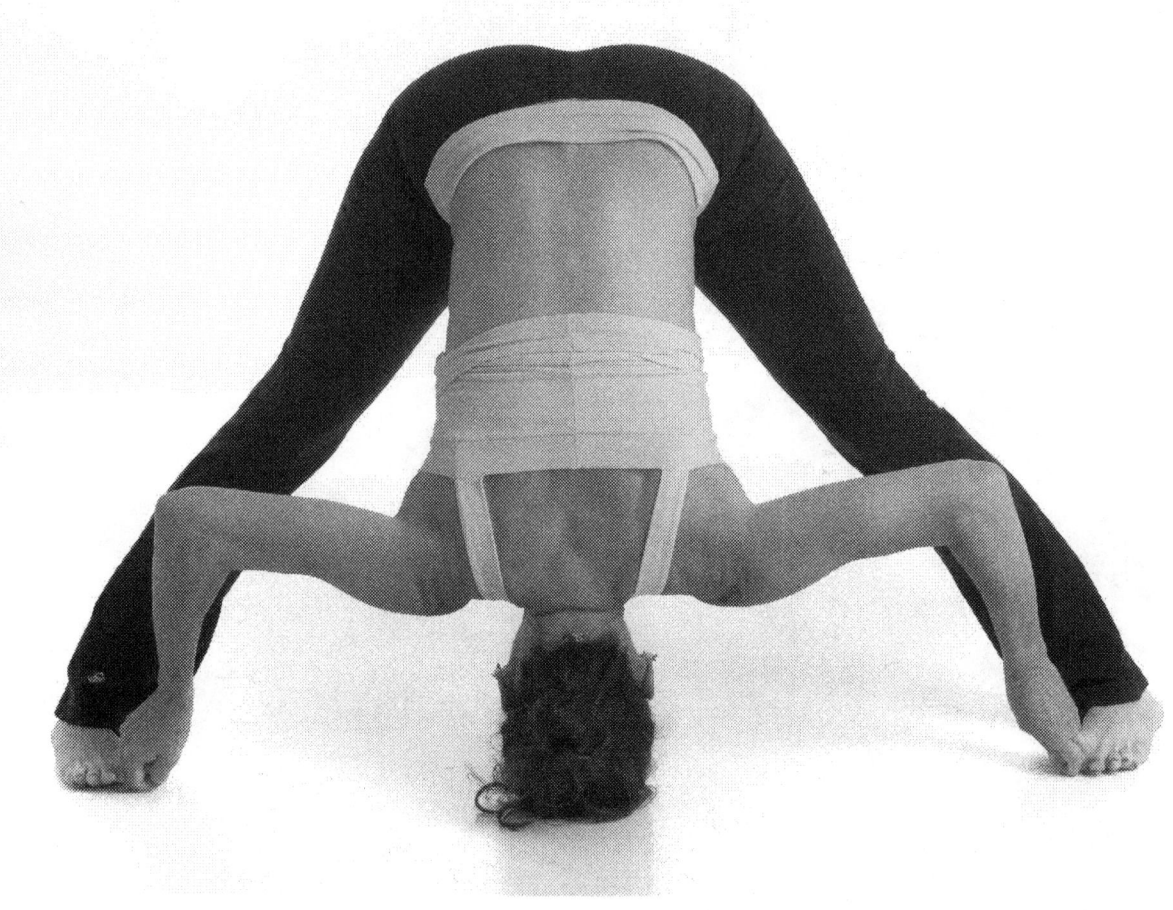

CHAKRA 2 SVADHISTHANA

This chakra is located behind the lower abdomen. The second chakra deals with sexuality and creativity issues. Do you have good healthy boundaries? Can you assert yourself? Do you take more or give more? Are you full of shame? Do you protect others, or do you need to be protected? Do you have control issues?

Organ Systems Impacted: *uterus, ovaries, vagina, cervix, testes, penis, bladder, large intestine, lower back*

Physical Dysfunctions: *fertility, urinary problems, sexual potency, pelvic and lower back pain, prostate and testicular disorders*

Yoga Posture: *Step into a wide stance with heels out and toes in, inhale deeply, exhale folding forward, inhale look up, grab toes with your first two fingers and thumb, or hands on knees, exhale drop your head.*

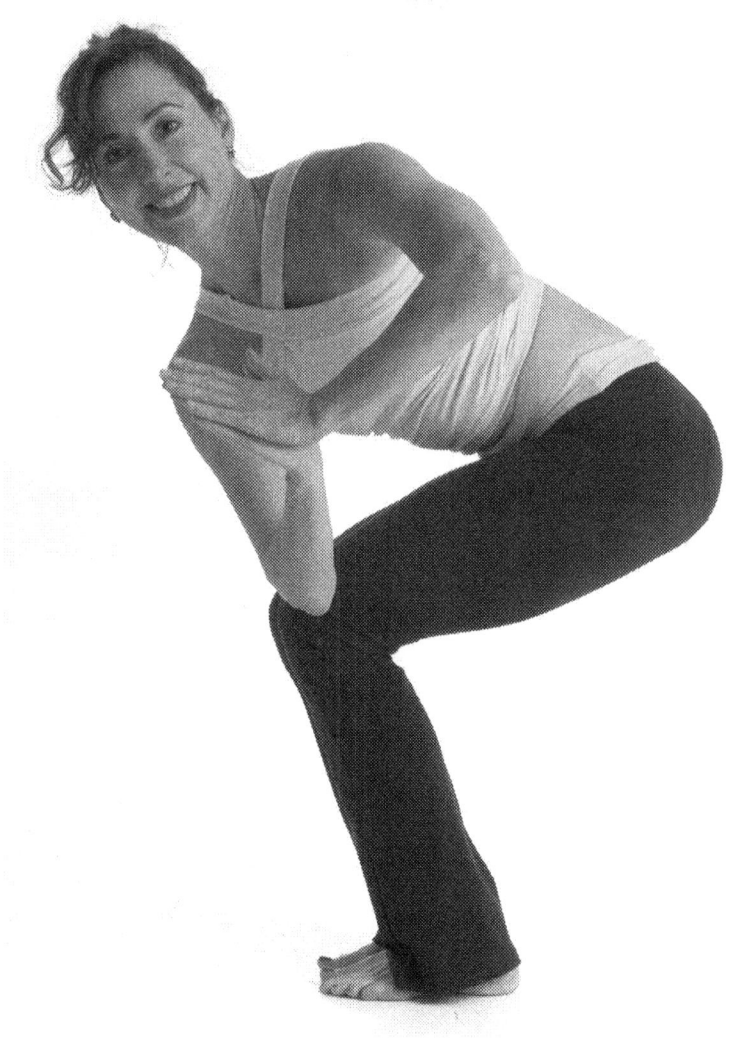

CHAKRA 3 MANIPURI

This chakra is located just above the belly button. It deals with the will or power. Are you comfortable with your own power? Are you competitive, or do you give up? Are you territorial? Are you responsible? Do you have addictions?

Organ Systems Impacted: *abdomen, upper intestines, liver, gallbladder, lower esophagus, stomach, kidney, pancreas, adrenal glands, spleen, middle spine*

Physical Dysfunctions: *diabetes, constipation and diarrhea, hepatitis, bulimia, anorexia nervosa, heartburn, gastritis, colon and intestinal problems, ulcerative colitis, duodenal ulcers*

Yoga Posture: *Place feet together, planted squarely on the floor, inhale deeply, exhale squat, press knees together, inhale, exhale drop opposite elbow to knee, twist looking over shoulder. Repeat on other side.*

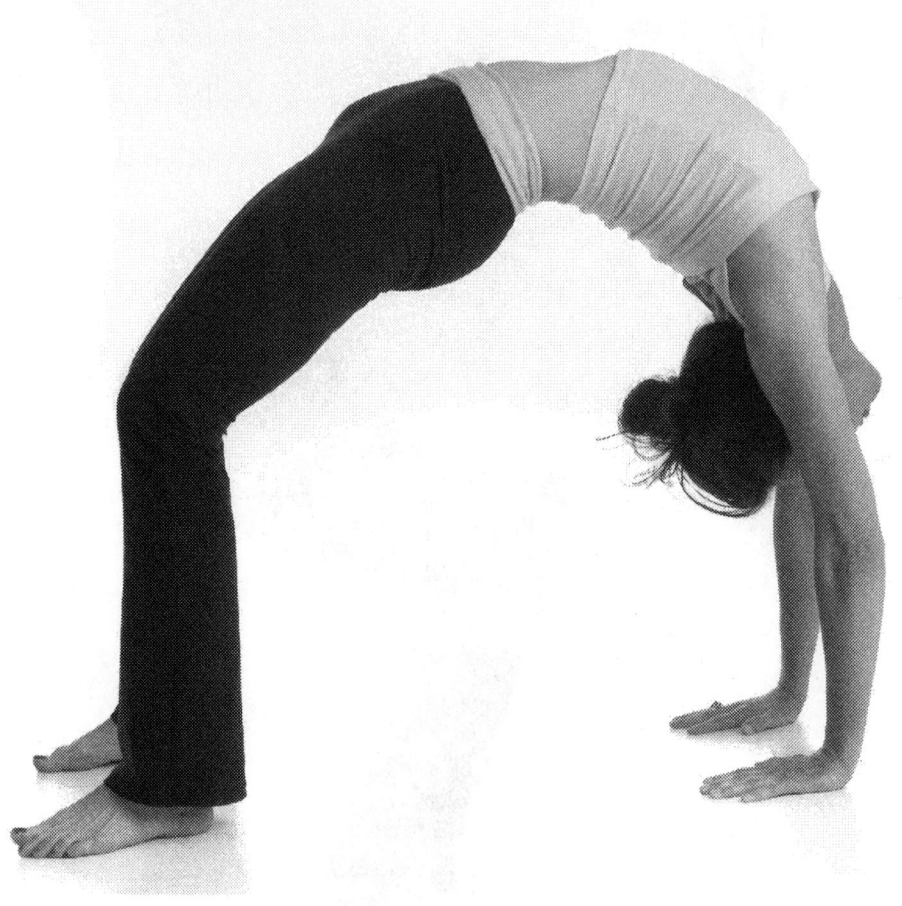

CHAKRA 4 ANAHATA

This is the heart chakra. It represents nurturing and emotional vulnerability. Can you feel love, and are you at peace with others? Do you have anger that's been suppressed? Can you forgive others, or do you hold grudges? Do you isolate yourself? Do you show courage and passion?

Organ Systems Impacted: *heart, lungs, blood vessels, shoulders, breasts, diaphragm, upper esophagus*

Physical Dysfunctions: *asthma, lung cancer, pneumonia, upper back problems, breast cancer, hypertension, chest pain, coronary disease*

Yoga Posture: *Beginners: lie on back, arms at your sides, bring feet to hips, inhale deeply, exhale lift hips with legs (bridge pose). Advanced: from bridge pose, place hands by shoulders, inhale, exhale come to top of head, straighten arms.*

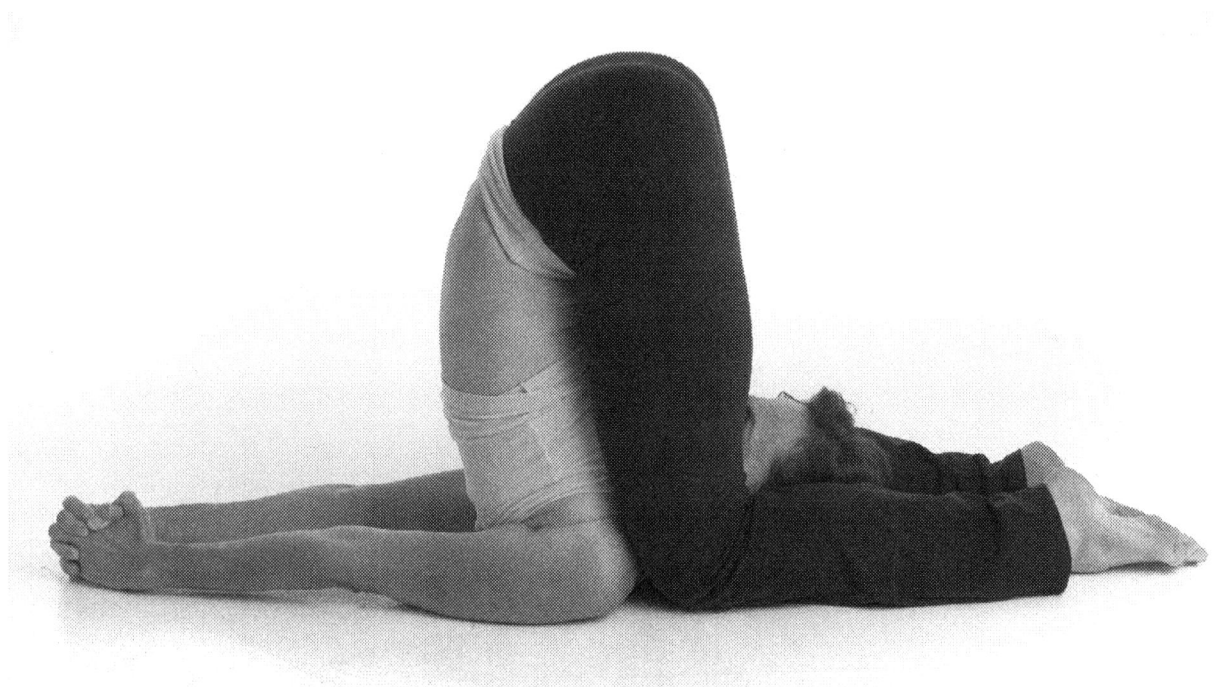

CHAKRA 5 VISUDDHU

This is the throat chakra, located at the base of the neck. It represents speaking your truth. Do you dominate others with your beliefs? Can you listen, or do you just talk? Do you have the patience to wait? Are you too stubborn to change your views?

Organ Systems Impacted: *thyroid, neck, mouth, jaw, teeth, throat*

Physical Dysfunctions: *Grave's disease, TMJ, cervical disk disease, hypothyroidism, bronchitis, mouth ulcers*

Yoga Posture: *Beginners: lie on back, inhale, exhale lift legs over head, place hands on hips for support, inhale, exhale drop feet over head, keep hands on hips. Advanced: inhale, exhale, drop knees to ground, clasp hands and extend arms.*

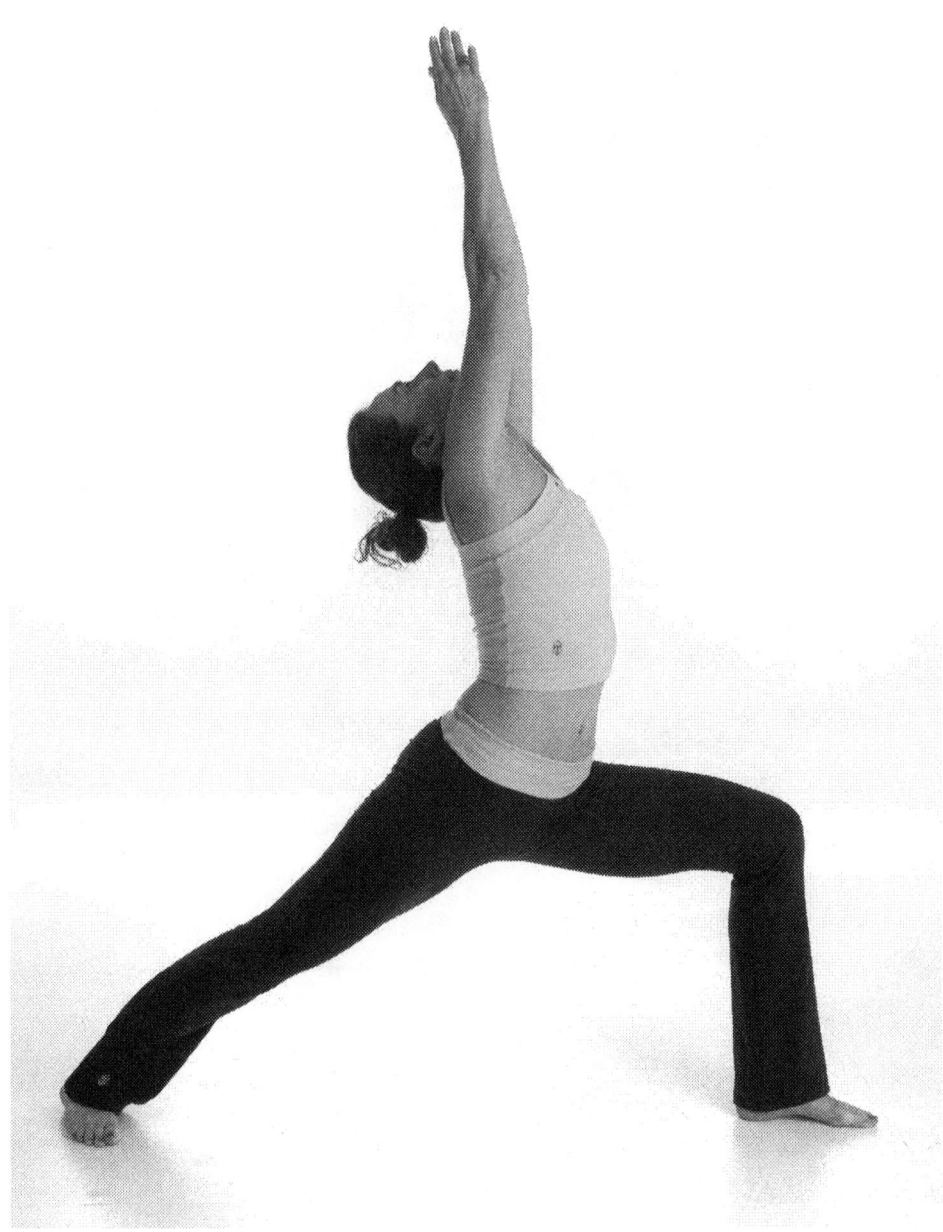

CHAKRA 6 AJNA

This chakra is located between the eyebrows. The third eye, or spiritual center, is another name for the sixth chakra. Do you have clarity in your life, and can you focus? Are you flexible or rigid? Are you critical in your thinking about yourself and others? Do you tend to think and not feel?

Organ Systems Impacted: *brain, eyes, ears, nose, pineal gland*

Physical Dysfunctions: *stroke, blindness, deafness, Parkinson's disease, learning disorders, neurological disturbances, brain tumors*

Yoga Posture: *Inhale, step legs 3½ feet apart, angle back foot 45°, turn toward front leg, exhale bend front leg, lift arms overhead. Repeat on other side.*

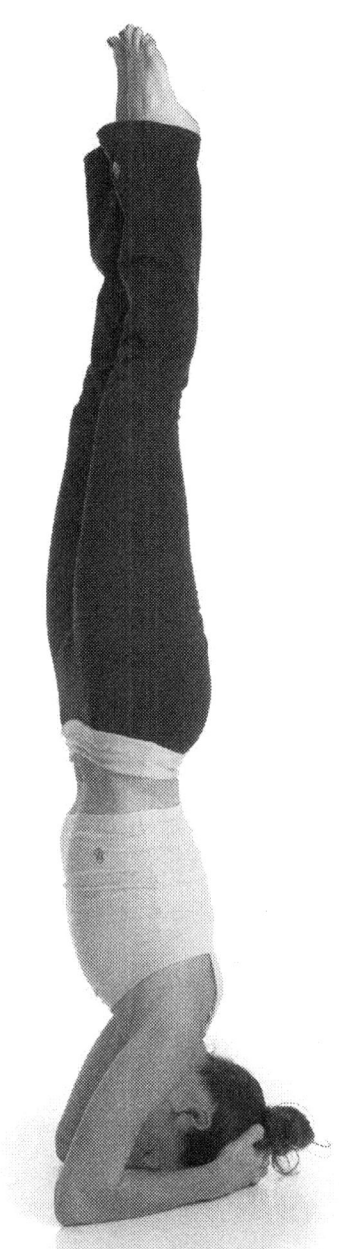

CHAKRA 7 SAHASRARA

This is the crown chakra, your connection to spirit. Do you know your life's purpose? Do you believe that you can influence events in your life? Do you have unhealthy attachments to this world?

Organ Systems Impacted: *any organ in your body*

Physical Dysfunctions: *any life threatening illness or accident, multiple systems abnormalities, lateral sclerosis, multiple sclerosis, genetic and developmental disorders*

Yoga Posture: *Beginners: inhale, exhale, kneel, place hands to elbows on floor then connect hands forming tripod, inhale, exhale place head in hands, straighten legs, lift hips. Advanced: lift legs into air*

A more playful and thought provoking way to learn about the chakras is through flower readings. I've worked with a local medical intuitive, Dr. Richard Jelusich, a gifted psychic, teacher and healer. A medical intuitive is a psychic who has the ability to visually scan a person's body and access an individual's health blueprint. I have hosted many flower reading dinner parties, to which my yoga students would bring a hand-picked flower. Before the feast would begin, Rick would close his eyes and, one by one, give each student a psychic reading based on the information he picked up from their flower. Rick would always share with my students what dominant chakra energy they were manifesting and any health problems they were experiencing, or going to experience, based on the chakra energy. He would then perform a spiritual physical healing.

A dinner of organic dishes would then follow the flower readings, as a way to continue the chakra discussion and ground each student back into the present moment. Both my students and I have benefited from this experience. Not only did the readings provide my students with more insight into themselves, but they provided me with more insight into my students, enabling me to be a better yoga teacher and healer for them. It turned out to be a very fun, informative and safe way to learn about chakras, yoga and our health.

Flower Reading and Dinner

Chilled Apple, Lemon and Ginger Elixir
Pan Seared Spicy Crab Cake on a Bed of Baby Greens
Herb Goat Cheese with Assorted Flat Breads
Red & Black Grapes

Butter Kissed Salmon with a Creamy Hummus & Raw Sprouted Salad
Mango Pineapple Salsa

Naughty White Chocolate Cheesecake
with Bosco Pears
and Sun Ripened Strawberry Sauce

Choice of Red or White Wine, Elan Specialty Coffee or Organic Green Tea

All foods are organic, blessed, and made with LOVE by Jyl

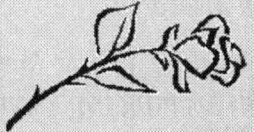

What chakra(s) address your health?

What chakra imbalances might you have?

What do you need to heal in your life?

Notes from Within: _____

_____
_____
_____
_____
_____
_____
_____
_____
_____
_____
_____
_____
_____
_____
_____
_____
_____
_____
_____
_____

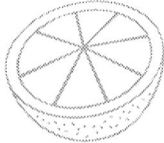

Doshas

Yoga is like going to church, having a therapy session and getting a physical healing all at the same time. Stay balanced!

A yogi can stay healthy by having balanced chakra energy. Another healing concept, and a great way to stay balanced, is to know your dosha. Doshas are a part of the Ayurvedic tradition. Ayurveda is a system of healing that originated in India and has been around for as long as yoga. During private sessions, I always encourage my students to discover their personal dosha. I briefly discuss the Ayurvedic ways of healing and how they relate to yoga. A dosha is your mind and body constitution. In other words, your dosha is your nature. Each one of us is born with a certain body type, with certain tendencies, certain limitations and certain ways we navigate the world.

Not only does each of us have our own personal dosha, but the world itself works by offering different doshas at different times of the day. In Ayurvedic medicine, the doshas are used extensively to heal, reconnect and balance people. It is believed that when the body is dis-at-ease with itself, or unbalanced, it becomes diseased. By knowing your own personal dosha, you can keep yourself from becoming sick. Understanding and practicing the doshas becomes a lifestyle, just like yoga. Like the chakras, there are specific yoga postures that heal certain doshas. To stay true to your dosha you must learn to go within.

THE FOUR DOSHAS

There are four doshas: Vatta, Pitta, Kapha and Tri-dosha. Each dosha gets its Sanskrit name from the language of the ancient Vedic civilization. The Vedic civilization developed the Ayurvedic system around 3000 B.C. The doshas represent elements in nature, with Vatta representing air and space, Pitta representing fire and water and Kapha representing earth and water. Tri-dosha represents all elements.

Before we go through each dosha in detail, please take the following test, so you can use it as a reference. Be honest in taking the test. Also, ask a spouse or someone who knows you really well to take the test for you. Check to see if you both come up with the same dosha. Enjoy yourself, but be careful, no cheating! Remember to honor your truth and have a little compassion toward yourself.

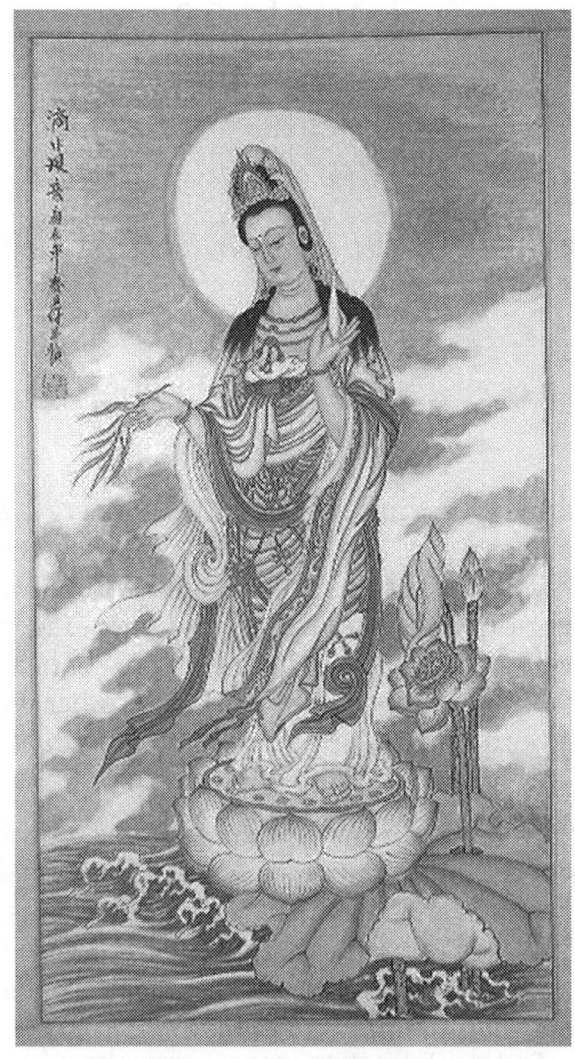

QUAN YIN: GODDESS OF COMPASSION

DISCOVERING YOUR MIND BODY TYPE

Instructions: The following questions are about you and your physical condition. Using the following scale, indicate how characteristic each statement is of you. There are no right or wrong answers, so answer each one as honestly as possible. Focus on general traits and characteristics which have been most prevalent in the past year. The following dosha test was taken from the Primordial Sound Meditation and Healing Workshop presented by the Chopra Center for Well Being.

	Not at all	Slightly	Somewhat	Moderately	Very
I tend to think and act quickly.	1	2	3	4	5
I learn new information quickly.	1	2	3	4	5
I am lively and enthusiastic by nature.	1	2	3	4	5
I tend to be thin and rarely gain weight.	1	2	3	4	5
My daily schedule of eating meals, going to sleep and awakening tends to vary.	1	2	3	4	5
Under stress, I tend to worry and become anxious.	1	2	3	4	5
I speak quickly and am a lively conversationalist.	1	2	3	4	5
My feet and hands tend to be cool.	1	2	3	4	5
I tend to have difficulty falling asleep.	1	2	3	4	5
My digestion tends to be irregular with frequent gas or bloating.	1	2	3	4	5
My hair tends to be on the dry side or kinky.	1	2	3	4	5
I have a low tolerance for cold weather.	1	2	3	4	5
I tend to eat quickly, finishing my meals before others at my table.	1	2	3	4	5
My skin tends to be dry.	1	2	3	4	5
My moods seem to change easily, and I tend to be sensitive and emotional.	1	2	3	4	5
Total for this section (Vatta): _____	_____	_____	_____	_____	_____

DISCOVERING YOUR MIND BODY TYPE

	Not at all	Slightly	Some-what	Moder-ately	Very
My skin is sensitive, sunburns or breaks out easily.	1	2	3	4	5
I have a tendency toward indigestion or heartburn.	1	2	3	4	5
I become uncomfortable in warm environments more readily than most people.	1	2	3	4	5
I tend to be a perfectionist with a low tolerance for errors.	1	2	3	4	5
My hair shows early thinning or graying or a tendency toward a reddish color.	1	2	3	4	5
It is not uncommon for me to have more than one bowel movement per day.	1	2	3	4	5
I sleep soundly and feel rested with less than eight hours of sleep.	1	2	3	4	5
I tend to perspire easily.	1	2	3	4	5
I think critically, am a good debater and can argue a point forcefully.	1	2	3	4	5
When pressured, I tend to become irritable and impatient.	1	2	3	4	5
If I begin a new project, I tend not to stop until I've completed it.	1	2	3	4	5
I have a strong appetite and can eat large quantities of food if I choose.	1	2	3	4	5
I tend to be strong-willed and somewhat forceful by nature.	1	2	3	4	5
I generally go over new information repeatedly until I am confident that I have mastered it.	1	2	3	4	5
I tend to perform my activities with precision and orderliness.	1	2	3	4	5
Total for this section (Pitta): _____	____	____	____	____	____

DISCOVERING YOUR MIND BODY TYPE

	Not at all	Slightly	Some-what	Moder-ately	Very
I am a good listener. I tend to speak only when I feel that I have something important to say.	1	2	3	4	5
I have a tendency to have chronic sinus congestion, asthma or excessive phlegm.	1	2	3	4	5
I sleep deeply for eight or more hours each night and get going slowly in the morning.	1	2	3	4	5
I have a slow digestion and tend to feel heavy after eating.	1	2	3	4	5
My hair tends to be thick, dark and wavy.	1	2	3	4	5
I tend to be sweet-natured and forgiving.	1	2	3	4	5
I generally don't enjoy climates that are cool, damp and cloudy.	1	2	3	4	5
I tend to eat slowly.	1	2	3	4	5
My skin is usually soft and smooth.	1	2	3	4	5
I tend to perform activities in a slow-paced manner.	1	2	3	4	5
It may take a while for me to learn something new, but once learned, I have good memory retention.	1	2	3	4	5
I tend to be loyal and devoted in my relationships.	1	2	3	4	5
I tend to gain weight easily and have difficulty losing extra pounds.	1	2	3	4	5
I tend to be steady and methodical with consistent energy and endurance.	1	2	3	4	5
I tend to be calm by nature and seldom lose my temper.	1	2	3	4	5
Total for this section (Kapha):____	____	____	____	____	____

VATTA_____   PITTA_____   KAPHA_____

TALLY UP YOU DOSHA SCORE

To find your dosha, add the columns in each section. Remember, for each column, add your total points. In other words, if you have circled four 5's, your total for that column is 20, not 4. Then add the column scores together for the total for that section.

Now that you have come up with a final count for each dosha, keep in mind that we are composed of all three doshas. Most of you will have one primary dosha. There will be a few who have scores with exactly the same number in each dosha. If you do, you folks are called Tri-doshas. This simply means that your mind-body makeup has been designed to have a balanced amount of all three doshas. It means that you are kept healthy by a number of different elements... Congratulations! But for the rest of us, we will have one primary and a secondary dosha to focus our attention on for our healing.

VATTA

Vattas physical characteristics are thin, light, active, quick, delicate and restless. Fashion models offer the best description of a Vatta's physical body. Vattas usually have a variable sex drive. They tend to be very mental and less physical. Vattas tend to be in more mentally stimulating careers and tend not to be athletic.

In general, Vattas welcome new experiences, hate life's routines, are lively conversationalists and spend money very easily. When Vattas are in balance, they are energetic, creative, adaptable, show initiative and are good communicators. But when Vattas are out of balance, or out of sync with life, they become mentally agitated, anxious, worried and are inconsistent and talkative. When they are out of balance, their digestive system becomes very delicate. When stress gets the best of Vattas, they tend to believe that they have done something to upset the situation and will blame themselves. Finally, Vattas are the ones that tend to forget all about food and the need to nourish their bodies. Count on a Vatta to forget to eat lunch.

PITTA

Pittas, on the other hand, will never forget lunch! They need a big meal to build their muscular bodies. Pittas are usually of medium build. They have very strong digestion and often need to eat lunch before noon. In fact, they are usually thinking about lunch at 10:00 a.m. Of all the doshas, Pittas do best as vegetarians. Their bodies are very warm, and they tend to perspire easily. Pittas tend to have reddish hair and light complexions. Athletic and competitive, they tend to be triathletes.

In general, Pittas have a sharp intellect and tend to be very direct and precise. They stay close to established routines and are great presenters and teachers. They love to spend money, usually on luxury items. When Pittas are in balance, they are bright, make good decisions and have a strong digestion. When they are out of balance, watch out! They get very angry and irritable and tend to be excessively critical and harsh, even aggressive and a bit intimidating. Under stress, Pittas will blame others, not themselves. As a yoga teacher, I need to know which students are my Pittas, because Pittas are the ones who will probably pass all edges in their yoga postures, get hurt and then possibly blame me for their injury! Who better to describe a Pitta, than a Pitta herself?

KAPHA

Kaphas tend to be big-boned with beautiful, clear smooth skin. They often have thick hair and sweet faces. Kaphas tend to move slowly and easily. They tend to hold on to their possessions. They are typically very solid individuals. Everyone should have a best friend that is a Kapha, as they are gentle, solid and wonderful to be around. Kaphas tend to gain weight very easily. It seems to them, by just looking at a piece of cake, they gain weight. For all their solidity, Kaphas need a personal coach or teacher to help them get started. I need to know the yoga students that are Kaphas, so I can help them move into their edge.

In general, Kaphas are easy going, have calm temperaments, are thoughtful, stable and devoted. Most Kaphas love to save money. When Kaphas are in balance they are steady, consistent, loyal, strong and supportive. When Kaphas are out of balance they are dull, inert, needy, attached, complacent and overly protective. But bless their hearts, when they are stressed to their limit, Kaphas, instead of casting blame, will ask how they can work with others to make the situation right.

FOODS

Foods that pacify the doshas are very important to know when you are trying to keep yourself balanced and healthy. There are six main groups of foods: sweet , sour, salty, pungent, bitter and astringent. The first is sweet foods. These foods are basic sugars of all kinds found in things like milk, butter, breads, rice, pasta and meats. Sour foods are the second group, and you might think of yogurt, lemon, tomatoes, sour fruits, vinegar and cheeses. Salty foods represent the next group, and these are any foods that contain salt. Pungent foods are considered spicy foods like ginger, hot pepper, cayenne pepper, garlic, radishes, chili peppers and cumin. Bitter foods are any of the leafy greens like romaine, endive, spinach, dandelion and arugula. This group also contains vegetables and turmeric spice. Finally, the last food group is astringent foods. Examples of this group are potatoes, broccoli, cauliflower, beans, lentils and pomegranates. I am sure you have foods in your own mind that you would consider for each group.

So considering the specific groups, let's look at each of the doshas. First, Vattas are pacified and balanced by sweet, sour and salty foods. If foods tend to be heavy, creamy, oily and served warm or hot, they will comfort Vattas when they are out of balance. Indian foods are my favorite when I need to soothe the Vatta in me. Also some Thai dishes help when a Vatta is out of balance and needs to be nurtured. I have a great Thai Coconut Salmon Curry dish that is a favorite and really works. Since most Vattas are slim, they can handle the calories. But for the Vattas that have lost their slim bodies, keep the calories low. Vattas with unhealthy living and eating habits will put on weight and should consider a dietary cleanse and new habits. Remember pungent, bitter and astringent foods will aggravate the Vatta body type, so it is best to avoid those foods.

Pittas are balanced by sweet, bitter and astringent foods. They should try to stay away from pungent, sour and salty foods. The heat of the day will really affect a poor Pitta, so they should eat cool foods. Smoothies work very well in balancing a Pitta who is overheated. A green salad with a piece of fish is a great lunch. I have found that in the morning, I can balance my Pitta by eating a cooling smoothie with my favorite fresh organic fruits and nuts. If you are cooking for a Pitta, remember to not make it too spicy. Most Pittas love their food spicy, but will pay because their digestive system is not set up to handle the extra heat. If you live with a Pitta and they get a little fired up, think cool foods.

Kaphas on the other hand, can eat spicy foods because they actually need to be stimulated a bit! My Kapha students love Mexican, Thai and Indian foods. My only concern for Kaphas is that they limit their intake. Kaphas need to keep an eye on the calories they are consuming, because they tend to hold onto things, including body fat. They are balanced by eating pungent, bitter and astringent types of foods. A cup of coffee (astringent) actually works to get them moving. Kaphas need to just say no to sweets. Yes, that would include desserts, pastas, breads and wine. Kaphas are aggravated by sweet, sour and salty foods. Remember Kaphas need extra support or coaching. Be kind to your Kapha friends and cook them light meals with small portion sizes. For dessert, try to encourage them to eat a piece of fruit. They will bless you for helping them to eat better and less.

To help you bring this healing concept into your life, every recipe will be labeled with symbols representing doshas. The symbols will help you see if the recipe is right for you. Don't worry, if your dominant dosha isn't on the dish, you can still enjoy it. Remember, we have all three doshas within us. Vattas look for the flower ❀, Pittas are the sun ☼, and Kaphas follow the snowflake ❄.

AYURVEDA DRINKS

PURIFICATION POTION ❀ ☼ ❄

Dates and almonds are considered to be sattvic (pure) and great for providing all doshas with increased energy.

> *4-5 raw dates (pitted)*
>
> *7-11 soaked raw almonds*
>
> *1 frozen banana*
>
> *½ cup coconut milk*
>
> *1 cup spring water*
>
> *1 cup organic soy milk or soy ice cream*

Soak dates and almonds overnight in water. In morning, pinch off and discard the almond skins. Add dates and almonds to banana, coconut milk, water and soy milk or ice cream, and puree in a blender.

TURMERIC TONIC ❀ ☼ ❄

Turmeric balances all three doshas. It helps to strengthen the digestion and purifies the blood. As a natural antibiotic, it protects intestinal flora.

> *1 teaspoon melted ghee (clarified butter, page 67)*
>
> *1 teaspoon turmeric*
>
> *1 cup soy milk*
>
> *1 tablespoon honey*
>
> *1 cup green or fruit tea*

Combine ingredients and heat.

ROSE MILKSHAKE ✿ ✩ ❄

This drink is cooling for Pittas, but good for all doshas. Rose petals nourish the heart and calm the mind.

> *2 tablespoons rose petal preserves (sold in most Indian food stores)*
>
> *2 cups soy milk or kefir (page 156)*
>
> *1 tablespoon spring water with three drops of rose essential oil (optional)*
>
> *1 cup frozen organic strawberries*

Using a mortar and pestle, reduce rose petals to a powder. If you prefer, you can use fresh petals from garden roses treated with organic fertilizers only. Combine powder with kefir, water and strawberries in a blender and puree. Garnish with a rose petal, and serve in a chilled glass.

SASSY SAFFRON COCKTAIL ✿ ✩ ❄

Saffron is known to revitalize the blood, the female reproductive system and the entire metabolism. This drink is great for all doshas.

> *1 cup of soy milk*
>
> *1 teaspoon saffron powder*
>
> *1 teaspoon melted ghee (page 67)*
>
> *honey or stevia (herbal sweetener) to taste*

Combine ingredients and serve warm in large mug, or over ice for a chilled delight. Use the honey to sweeten a hot drink, and stevia for the cold version.

WARM ALMOND, CARDAMOM AND NUTMEG BREW ❄

This brew will pacify Kaphas. Cardamom is one of the best digestive stimulants. When added to milk it neutralizes its mucus-forming properties and brings life-force prana into the body.

> *10-15 soaked raw almonds*
>
> *1 cup purified water*
>
> *1 cup milk (or milk substitute)*
>
> *1 teaspoon ground cardamom*
>
> *1 teaspoon ground nutmeg*
>
> *1 teaspoon rose water*
>
> *honey to taste*

Soak almonds for eight hours in purified water and drain. Pinch skins off almonds and discard. Combine almonds and water and blend. In a heavy saucepan, combine almond mixture and milk. Add cardamom, nutmeg, rose water and honey, heat and serve warm.

DOSHA WORKOUT

Not only do foods play a huge part in keeping the doshas healthy, exercise is also a key component to creating a healthy mind-body constitution. All doshas will benefit from yoga and meditation. Vattas require yoga and meditation in their lives to keep their active minds quiet and peaceful. Because their frames are more delicate, they will also benefit from lighter workouts such as swimming, walking, dance, golf, martial arts, horseback riding, tennis, baseball, bicycling and Pilates.

Pittas on the other hand, need more demanding exercise. Because of their aggressive nature, they need an intense workout. Think of Pittas as being triathletes. Balancing sports for them are basketball, cycling, diving, ice skating, rowing/kayaking, mountain biking, sailing, skiing, surfing, wind surfing and touch football. Remember, Pittas love cold climate sports. If you are thinking about going to the snow and you need a friend to go with… avoid Vattas and Kaphas… ask a Pitta.

Kaphas, in spite of their placid and noncompetitive natures, are born athletes. They may be late bloomers in regard to knowing their athletic abilities. They tend to be the chubby children that get ignored. They may need a coach or personal trainer to push them into their physical realm, but when they "grow up," they often become professional athletes. Sports that keep them in balance are hard-core aerobics, basketball, body building, calisthenics, cross-country running and skiing, lacrosse, javelin, gymnastics, fencing, cycling, rowing, racquetball, rock climbing, sculling, soccer and volleyball.

DOSHA TIME

It is exciting to know the world works on the dosha system too! Certain hours during the day are considered to be specific dosha times. For instance, from 6:00 a.m. to 10:00 a.m. is considered Kapha time. Isn't it just about that time of day, you reach for a cup of coffee to get you moving? This time of day brings out the Kapha in all of us, and we need a little jump-start. The best jump-start is a morning workout program. This is the best time of day to workout, because our muscles and joints can safely handle resistance.

10:00 a.m. to 2:00 p.m. is Pitta time. This is the best time for all of us to EAT. Remember, Pittas have the best digestion systems. At this time of day, we all can handle incoming food. Eat and be happy! You should eat your largest meal at this time of day. People who skip lunch during this hour and eat big dinners are likely to be overweight.

From 2:00 p.m. to 6:00 p.m. is Vatta time. This is the best time of the day for all of us to be mentally stimulated. If you need to be creative, work on it at this time of day. So sit down, and let the creative juices flow.

From 6:00 p.m. to 10:00 p.m. is Kapha time again. At this time of day, don't you feel like you can just go to bed? The body is indeed preparing for sleep. So avoid starting any projects. Learn to let the body slow down. This is the best time to go to sleep.

If you stay up past 10:00 p.m., you have just gone into Pitta time and will probably start to get hungry again. I know many people who say they are night owls and stay up late. Many of these people are overweight. During Pitta time you will get a second wind, and it will seem like you are a night owl. But trust me; this is hard on the body. The body actually needs you to be asleep during this hour so it can do its job and digest the food from the day. Most people who stay up will start to eat more food. Now the body is forced to stop the purification process to handle more incoming food.

Have you ever awoken at 2:00 a.m. with too much on your mind? Welcome to Vatta time. From 2:00 a.m. to 6:00 a.m. is the best time to get up. This is also a great time to write, meditate, or do yoga. I often get up at this time of day and feel that it is truly a magical time. Between the hours of 4:00 a.m. and 6:00 a.m., your entire glandular system can be regulated by meditation. By regulating glandular secretions in the proper amounts, you actually create healthier blood chemistry.

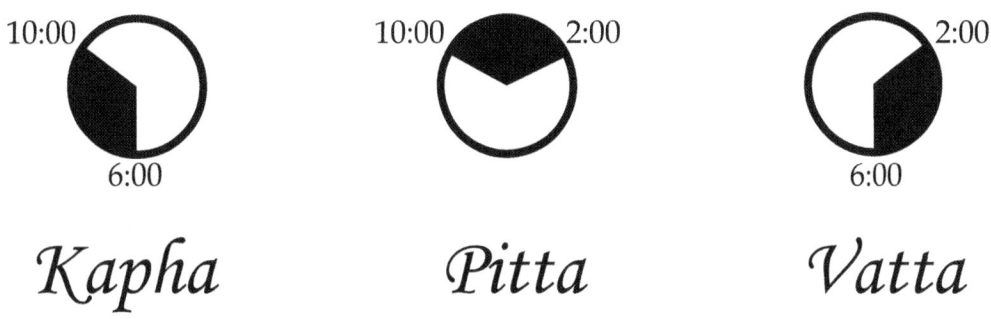

If you think about it, we put our children to sleep according to the dosha system. The healthy way to live is to go to sleep when the sun goes down and rise with the sun. Remember the saying, "early to bed, early to rise"… something about "healthy, wealthy, and wise"…. Try living your life by the dosha times, and see the difference it can make in your life and health. After one of my first dosha workshops, one of my students started following this practice. He said he noticed a huge difference in how he felt.

ESSENTIAL OILS

Every night after yoga and before dinner, I give my students an aromatherapy head and foot massage. I use an essential oil around their heads and discuss the properties of it, as they are rolling up their mats and laying out their blankets and eye pillows. I want them to learn about the oils and their healing properties, so they will feel comfortable using them on their own at home.

So many students ask me how to use essential oils. I always tell them if it smells good, then it is the right oil. Find your dosha and see if you agree with the matching oils. This is a great reference for when you are having one of those down days. Put a couple of drops of oil in the palm of your hand. Rub your hands together, smell the oil and apply it to your body. Go within to ask your body where to place the oil. Now you are good to go! When it comes to the oils, remember less is more. Just a couple of drops, and if you are sensitive, please dilute with your favorite massage oil.

VATTA IMBALANCE

Clary Sage	Basil	Juniper Berry
Frankincense	Lavender	Lemongrass
Sandalwood	Ginger	Eucalyptus

PITTA IMBALANCE

Yarrow	Lemon	Angelica
Spearmint	Jasmine	Musk
Peppermint	Rose	Cedarwood

KAPHA IMBALANCE

Eucalyptus	Cloves	Orange
Fennel	Bayberry	Hibiscus
Cinnamon	Nutmeg	Myrrh

From Egyptian hieroglyphics and Chinese manuscripts, we know priests and physicians have been applying oils directly to the skin for healing purposes for thousands of years. Essential oils are the volatile liquids that are distilled from plants. These high vibrating substances heal and add vitality to the body. Also consider using oils in your food. In the following chapter's love rose sauce, I use a couple of drops of rose oil.

One of my favorite brands of essential oils is Young Living. They use the most sophisticated methods of distilling the oils, creating very high quality healing oils. You won't find these oils in your local health food store, as they are a direct supplier.

I was traveling in Central America this year, and during the trip I used essential oils. Every day, I would get up and apply five different oils. One day, I noticed mosquitoes were attacking everyone in my group. By the end of the day, most of the group had ugly boils on their skin from the attacks. I found that not one mosquito came my way that day, most likely because of the essential oils. So, if you are traveling, always bring your favorite essential oils with you.

BENEFITS OF ESSENTIAL OILS

Greatly enhance the immune system

Absorb quickly into every cell of the body within 20 minutes

They are metabolized like other nutrients

They are powerful antioxidants, with anti-bacterial, anti-parasitic, anti-cancerous, anti-fungal, anti-infectious, anti-tumor and antiseptic properties

Help remove metallic particles and toxins from the air

Increase atmospheric oxygen

Destroy odors from mold, cigarettes and animals

Help promote emotional, physical and spiritual healing

SOME COMMON OILS AND THEIR USES

OIL	USES
Basil	Alleviates mental fatigue
Bergamot	Helps to relieve anxiety
Birch	Helps with arthritis; also a lymphatic cleanse
Clary Sage	Promotes estrogen balance in the tissues
Clove	Anti-bacterial, anti-fungal, anti-infectious, a strong antiseptic
Cypress	Decongestant and very relaxing
Eucalyptus	Great for coughs and colds
Frankincense	Oxygenates the pineal and pituitary glands
Geranium	Helps balance the hormones
Grapefruit	Anti-depressant

SOME COMMON OILS AND THEIR USES

OIL	USES
Jasmine	Promotes a feeling of confidence
Juniper	Evokes feelings of health, love and peace
Lavender	Balancing and calming; healing for all skin conditions
Lemongrass	Helps improve circulation
Myrrh	Helps to heal chapped or cracked skin and reduce inflammation
Nutmeg	Supports the adrenal glands for increased energy
Orange	Brings about peace and happiness
Patchouli	Protection from UV radiation and tightens skin; reduces wrinkles
Peppermint	Stimulates the nerves; great for sore muscles
Rose	Revitalizing and rejuvenating; great anti-depressant
Sandalwood	Powerfully calms and focuses the body; great for yoga and meditation
Spruce	Helps release emotional blocks
Ylang Ylang	Stimulating and balancing to energies; creates peacefulness

What is your dosha?

How can you support and balance your dosha?

Which essential oils do you gravitate toward?

Notes from Within: _____

_____
_____
_____
_____
_____
_____
_____
_____
_____
_____
_____
_____
_____
_____
_____
_____
_____
_____
_____
_____
_____

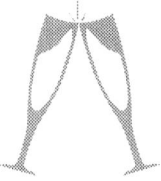

Yoga and Dinner

Now that you have finished your private yoga session, you are invited to attend Yoga and Dinner by Jyl.

Cooking with Love and Reckless Passion

Have you ever eaten food that looks beautiful, but is missing something? Usually that missing something is LOVE. I know when a chef in a restaurant is having a bad day. I can taste it, and I can feel the food is missing a higher vibration. I try to ground myself and say a prayer to God before I start cooking. Then I turn up the music and rock out in the kitchen. I always Reiki the food I serve. Reiki is accessing healing energy from the universe. A Reiki Master can initiate anyone into the Reiki healing system. I recommend it to all. I focus on loving thoughts as I am cooking. I encourage all my students to cook. So let's step into the kitchen together and start preparing for our own yoga and dinner party.

Getting Started

For starters, bring love into your kitchen. Open your heart to your partner, your children, your friends and most importantly to yourself. Find ways to nurture that passion in your kitchen spiritually, physically and emotionally. This might even mean having sex in your kitchen! You will begin to cook the most beautiful dishes, with lots of passion and with all your heart. Fear keeps many out of the kitchen. So I challenge you all to start cooking from the heart. At its best, preparing food should be an act of love, not drudgery. A big fancy kitchen is not required. Some of my most wonderful dishes were created in a small kitchen. Sometimes there may not have been a lot in the refrigerator, other than lots of love and leftover passion.

Learn to create love everyday!!!! Life is short. Eat, drink and fall in love.

THE LOVE ROSE SAUCE WITH CHICKEN BREAST ❁ ✿ ❊

Roasted Free-Range Chicken

6 breasts free-range chicken

4 cloves garlic, crushed

1 teaspoon sea salt

4 tablespoons (½ stick) organic butter

½ cup organic free-range chicken stock

¼ cup fresh lemon juice

Set oven to 375° F. Rub chicken with salt, garlic and butter. Place chicken in a roasting pan, add stock and juice, roast for 30 minutes. Let chicken cool.

Love Rose Sauce

12 red organic roses (petals)

12 organic dry chestnuts

2 teaspoons butter or ghee (page 67)

4 drops rose oil (Young Living oil)

2 tablespoons ground anise

2 tablespoons honey

1 papaya, chopped

2 cups red wine

As the chicken is roasting, use a mortar and reduce rose petals for sauce. Follow the directions on the package for roasting organic chestnuts, and make a paste. Combine roses, chestnut paste, butter or ghee, rose oil, anise, honey, garlic and papaya in a saucepan. Cook over medium heat and slowly add wine.

I thinly slice the chicken and add it to the sauce. The chicken takes on a reddish color, and your guests (other yogis) might think they are eating red meat. When serving the dish, drizzle the rose sauce over the chicken, and garnish with a small white rose. Serves six.

One of the nicest comments I heard from a student about Yoga and Dinner, was that it inspired her to go back to her kitchen and cook in a new way for her family. Their dinners went from a free-for-all situation, with each person grabbing whatever they wanted, to actually sitting down at a candlelit table and sharing a beautiful healthy organic meal. The nightly dinner soon became a familial celebration, with everyone opening their hearts.

HOW TO CREATE YOUR OWN YOGA AND DINNER PARTY

Set a date and invite all your favorite yogis (or potential yogis!).

Design your menu. Make sure you mindfully set a menu that can be enjoyed by all of your guests.

Clear your living room or another large room in your house of all furniture.

Make sure you have plenty of candles to light.

Prepare the menu in the morning. Foods should all be ready to just heat and serve.

Have water goblets ready with water and garnish. I usually use herbs from my garden, like a snippet of lavender with a slice of lime.

Have the silverware wrapped in linen napkins, tied with beautiful fabric or ribbons. Sometimes, for special events, I will put a beautiful hand written saying or quote on a small piece of paper and attach it to the napkin by the ribbon.

Have your favorite yoga teacher scheduled to come by at 6:30 p.m. to teach the class. There are many yoga teachers who would be honored to come to your home, including this one!

Pick soothing, meditative music to create a relaxing mood. I love Deva Premal's music when I can't have live music. There are so many artists out there… support them and let them play for dinner.

Offer yoga props, such as eye pillows, belts, bolsters and blankets.

Have your guests bring wine or anything their hearts desire. I had one woman treat her friends to new yoga clothing.

Yoga and Dinner is a great girls, couples and family night out.

YOGA AND DINNER SCHEDULE

6:30 guided meditation lying down with eyes closed

6:45 begin yoga asana practice

7:45 seated meditation

7:50 rest pose; foot and head massage; take turns with each other or invite your favorite massage therapist

8:00 wake up the yogis and serve dinner

Warning: After several Yoga and Dinner sessions, you may have a hard time going to a studio to do yoga. Once you create a sacred place in your home and start doing yoga, you will notice a change. Your house will never be the same. When people walk into my sacred space they feel the love immediately. It's like yoga is in the walls.

A Favorite Yoga by Jyl Dinner

Thai Coconut Curried Salmon with Greens

Fresh Garden Vegetables

Brown Basmati Rice

Tofu Cake with Chocolate Ganache Sauce

Fresh Strawberries and Mint Leaf Garnish

Drizzled with Chocolate

Red or White Wine

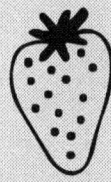

THAI COCONUT CURRIED SALMON WITH GREENS

This is a favorite of most my students!

1 pound wild salmon fillet, skinned
2 tablespoons ghee or butter
1 cup thinly sliced onion
½ teaspoon red curry paste
1-14oz can light coconut milk
2 tablespoons curry powder
1 tablespoon maple syrup
2 tablespoons lime juice
1 tablespoon minced fresh ginger
1 tablespoon fish sauce
2 teaspoons minced garlic
1-8oz bottle clam juice
6 cups watercress or spinach

1. Cook the salmon separately in a medium saucepan. Place enough purified water to cover fish and bring to a boil. Poach the salmon for 10 minutes. The fish will start to have cooked edges. Flip salmon and turn off heat. If you forgot to buy skinned salmon, this is a good time to remove the skin and discard. Let the fish continue to cook in the saucepan while you are making the curry.

2. In a separate saucepan, heat ghee or butter over medium-high heat and add onions and curry powder. Cook until tender, about 10 minutes.

3. Add coconut milk, curry paste, maple syrup, lime juice, ginger, fish sauce, garlic and clam juice to the skillet and continue to cook on low heat.

4. Using your hands, pull the salmon apart into bite sized pieces and add to the curry. Right before serving, add greens and heat. Serve warm with brown rice or quinoa. Garnish with your favorite lightly sautéed vegetables.

JYL'S FAMOUS TOFU BIRTHDAY CAKE

2 ¼ cups oat flour
2 teaspoons baking powder
½ teaspoon sea salt
1 ¼ cups sucanat sugar
½ cup butter, room temperature
7 ounces soft tofu
1 ½ cups soy milk
2 teaspoons vanilla
½ cup strawberry jam
1 pint fresh organic strawberries, thinly sliced

1. Preheat oven to 350°F. Grease two 8-inch cake pans.
2. In a large bowl, combine oat flour, baking powder and salt. Set aside.
3. In another bowl, mix sugar and butter until creamy.
4. In a food processor or blender, mix tofu, soy milk and vanilla until smooth. Combine tofu and sugar mixtures. Add liquid mixture to dry ingredients.
5. Pour batter into pans and bake for 30 minutes.
6. Cool cakes to room temperature. Place one cake layer on serving plate and evenly spread strawberry jam and fresh sliced strawberries on top. Place second cake layer over first and frost with chocolate ganache sauce.

CHOCOLATE GANACHE SAUCE

1 cup heavy cream or soy milk
1 package semisweet chocolate chips or tofu chocolate chips

1. Combine liquid and chips in a double boiler and melt.
2. Stir mixture until fully melted and smooth.
3. Drizzle chocolate in middle of cake and let drip down the sides.

PRESENTATION IS EVERYTHING... How you serve your food and how you present yourself is all influenced by the thoughts you have in your head and the core of your essence. Yoga helps you learn to let your light shine.

How can you bring love into your kitchen?

Notes from Within: _____

Design your own yoga and dinner party.

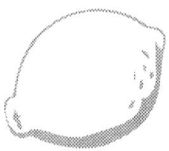

Begin Healing with Foods

The more yoga (and yoga dinners!) you enjoy, and the better you eat, the more you will start to feel and look great. Yes - you may even start to lose weight!

We have created a fast world and fast food to match our pace. We have created a world full of cell phone zombies, addicted to Palm Pilots and BlackBerrys. We have created a world where we have all the conveniences, yet it is my belief that it is not to our highest purpose and our best health. I spend a lot of time asking WHY? Why do we create processed foods that are convenient, but could cause possible pain and sickness? We eat mindlessly, usually whatever we can get our hands on at the time. Then off we go to our health care system when our bodies stop supporting us. Our western system of medicine is set up to treat our symptoms, and when that symptom is a broken arm or a ruptured spleen, it usually does a good job. But too many of our ailments are treated by prescribing expensive drugs that often create unhealthy side effects. We don't allow our bodies to heal themselves. In fact, we get in the way. WHY? Why aren't we producing foods that heal our bodies? Why are we not honoring the foods that God gave us to eat for proper health? I truly don't want genetically designed foods or foods sprayed with harmful toxins. I want the food that my grandpa grew in healthy soil and with love.

I was on a flight headed to Ohio and picked up an in-flight magazine. I opened the magazine to an article entitled "Where's the Fat? Trans fat may not be on the label, but you can bet it's clogging your arteries right now." The FDA estimates that by 2009, the cases of coronary heart disease and annual deaths will decline substantially, simply by listing the bad fats on food labels. Trans fats, or man made fats, are in everything from cookies and salty snacks to wheat thins and microwave popcorn. The FDA estimates that 40 percent of all food on grocery store shelves contains some trans fat. Starting in the year 2006, the FDA will require all food labels to list the trans fats, or bad fats. These fats include hydrogenated oil, partially hydrogenated oil and vegetable shortening.

As I looked around at the food being served on the flight, I could not help but notice the label; no mention of trans fats. If you pay attention to the total grams of fat that are listed on labels, you will notice that sometimes it doesn't add up. Take the total fat grams, subtract the listed fat grams, and the remaining grams are trans fat. I wanted to tell the unsuspecting guy seated next to me not to eat his breakfast bar, because the bar contained 45 grams of trans fats, but I just kept it to my healthy self. For the record, I would not dream of eating airline food. I have done so much healing and yoga, I find it is extremely hard to eat out anywhere. I have learned to pack my food and choose my restaurants carefully.

I will never forget when I was with my mother in her hospital room, supporting her as she was trying to recover from a serious illness. When lunch was served, I nearly went through the ceiling. My sick mother was served potato chips, canned tomato juice, a ham and cheese sandwich, coffee and ice cream. All these foods were processed and laden with unhealthy fats and sodium. My mother's body was already so swollen from the over use of prescription drugs for her fibromyalgia; how was her body going to heal itself with processed foods and trans fats? When are we going to wake up and demand better food? When are we going to demand foods that can truly heal us?

> **FOOD MYTH**: Saturated fats are BAD. **TRUTH**: Saturated fats are fine in moderation. My Grandfather lived into his 90's eating lard every day. Stay away from trans fats. Research now shows that it is the lack of omega 3 fats in our diets that causes high unhealthy levels of cholesterol.

My clients often ask me about the trendy high protein diets, South Beach diets, low carbohydrate diets and sexy super food diets. The first question I ask them is, "Does that feel right?" Many of them have no idea what I am talking about. If I put bad food in my mouth, I almost immediately get sick for hours. I realize that not everyone is as sensitive to foods as I am, but all of us have an internal intelligence when it comes to healthy food choices. So, instead of telling a student which trendy diet to follow, I try to help them discover and reconnect with their own internal voice.

When the body does a lot of yoga, it needs healthier foods. My regular yoga students get very sensitive to foods. I did have one student, who hasn't devoted much time to yoga, tell me that he was not about to restrain himself from eating unhealthy foods that brought him pleasure. I told him that a regular diet of these foods, like cakes, cookies, snacks and fried foods could some day bring him disease. I also told him to keep up with his yoga, and he would come to discover his own truth. When you are at a higher level of consciousness and healing, you are going to gravitate toward foods that are good for you. I suggest the following list for conscious eating.

TIPS ON EATING TO HEAL

1. Eat organic foods whenever possible. Studies have shown that organically grown produce can contain 300% more minerals and total nutritional value than commercially grown produce. Good health cannot be maintained without an adequate supply of minerals.

2. Stay away from ALL processed foods.

3. Ask your favorite restaurants to start using organic foods and healthy fats and oils.

4. Understand food combining. Refer to "The Body Ecology Diet" by Donna Gates. She explains how to avoid combining foods that may harm your digestion. For example, refrain from eating grains with proteins… and yes, that would mean that you don't eat an American sandwich. Eat fruits by themselves.

5. Eat for your dosha. Notice if you feel better when you pick foods that support your mind-body design.

6. Replace table salt with organic Celtic Sea salt or kosher salt. Celtic Sea salt offers the highest level of minerals to your diet.

7. Try eating for your blood type. Follow the suggestions in "Cook Right for Your Type" by Dr. Peter J. D'Adamo.

8. For high heat cooking, use ghee (purified butter), unrefined coconut oil, lard or butter (saturated fats) sparingly. Unrefined Coconut oil is excellent for the thyroid. Use Olive oil (monounsaturated fat) in salad dressings.

> **RECIPE FOR MAKING YOUR OWN GHEE**
> Heat one pound of organic butter in a saucepan on low heat. The butter will start to separate as it melts. Skim off the milky white residue and discard. Store ghee, clarified butter, in a cool dry place.
> Easy!

9. Stay away from trans fats, partially hydrogenated oil, hydrogenated oil, vegetable shortening, soybean oil and margarine. These oils can contribute to the development of cancer, heart disease and many other health concerns.

10. Grind flax seeds just before using them instead of using flax seed oil, which can be unstable.

11. Eat wild salmon instead of farmed salmon. Eat hormone-free meats and poultry.

12. Do eat eggs… brown eggs, fertile eggs, free range eggs, omega 3 eggs and organic eggs… they are all good!

13. Stay away from all salad dressing unless you made it yourself.

14. Try sprinkling wheat germ on top of smoothies, salads and steamed vegetables.

15. Eat at home more or pack your lunch, so you know exactly what you are eating.

16. Try to eliminate sugar, caffeine (yes, that would include chocolate) and alcohol from your diet. You will gradually start to feel better and your moods will stabilize. If you need caffeine to get you going in the morning, green tea, which is high in antioxidants, is a great substitute for your morning coffee.

17. Stay hydrated by drinking at least 8 glasses of water a day.

18. Stay away from the Standard American Diet… SAD… play around with your own likes and dislikes. Pay attention to how you feel after you eat. Eat foods that make you feel good. Remember, the purer you get, the more you will understand what I mean.

19. Always sit and honor the food you eat. After a big meal, try lying down on the floor on your left side for ten minutes to ensure proper digestion. Turmeric is a spice that can aid with digestion. I always put a little in my tea after a meal.

20. Avoid processed white breads and flour products. If you have a problem with yeast, try eliminating it from your meals. Eat organic sprouted whole grain breads without yeast that are wheat-free.

21. Try juicing with fresh organic vegetables and fruits.

22. Replace your sugar with stevia, an herbal sweetener. Eat more fruits when you are craving sweets.

23. Replace some of your old favorites, like yogurt, with something new, like kefir. You can learn more about kefir on page 156. In addition to eating kefir, I take a probiotic every morning and in the evening before bed. Both are very good for the colon and help to replenish the good bacteria.

24. Balance your intake of acid foods with alkaline foods. An alkaline body is a healthy body. Look at your food before you put it into your mouth. Does 20% of your meal come from acid-forming foods and 80%, or the rest of the food on your plate, from an alkaline source? This is key, because a diseased body is an acid body. A tip on staying alkaline is to add Supergreens into your daily drinking water. You can find Supergreens at any health food store. I also add a couple drops of liquid mint chlorophyll, which helps to purify the blood.

MAINTAINING AN ALKALINE BODY

ACID FOODS	ALKALINE FOODS
Alcohol	All fresh fruits
Black pepper and salt	All raw vegetables
Bottled salad dressings	All salad greens
Breads	All sprouts
Cakes and cookies	Apple cider vinegar (raw)
Canned and frozen foods	Appreciation
Chocolate	Dates
Cigarettes	Dried apricots
Coffee	Dried figs
Complaining	Dulse (ocean vegetable)
Cooked grains, except millet and quinoa	Fresh or dried seasoning herbs
Dairy	Fresh, raw juices
Distilled vinegar	Fun
Eggs	Grapefruit (but do not mix with other foods)
Foods cooked in oils	Herbal teas
Fruits that have been glazed or sulfured	Honey
Meat, fish, poultry and shellfish	Joy
Nuts, seeds and legumes	Maple syrup
Pasta	Melon (but do not mix with other foods)
Popcorn	Millet
Processed cereals	Molasses
Processed foods with wheat or white flour	Lima beans
Processed milks (soy, rice, almond)	Potatoes
Soda crackers	Positive thinking
Soft drinks	Quinoa

MAINTAINING AN ALKALINE BODY

ACID FOODS	ALKALINE FOODS
Sugar	Raisins
Sulking	Raw, cold pressed olive oil (organic)
Tea (except herbal, caffeine free tea)	Raw, cold pressed flax seed oil
Tofu and soy products	Supergreens

25. Eat more sprouted seeds, grains and beans. Soaking and sprouting offers you more nutrients. Sprouting also eliminates certain acids and toxins that could interfere with digestion. Most health food stores carry sprouts, or you can learn to make them yourself. Remember to start out with the living raw form. Soaking is done by placing the seeds, grains or beans in a glass container of purified water. The container can sit on your kitchen counter top while soaking. Sprouting occurs after the soaking process. Place the plant in a colander and drain off water. Each plant is rinsed daily. Sprouting will occur at different times. Quinoa takes one day to sprout while chickpeas sprout in 2-3 days. After the plants start to sprout, refrigerate them. Sprouts are good for 3 days.

DO IT YOURSELF SPROUTS

PLANTS	SOAKING TIME	SPROUTING TIME
Almonds	8 hours	no sprouting
Chickpeas	8 hours	2-3 days
Flax seeds	1/2 hour	no sprouting
Quinoa	2 hours	1 day
Lentil	7 hours	3 days
Sunflower seeds	6 hours	2 days

JUICING...

In California, it is not unusual to see people drinking shots of wheatgrass or juicing to get their nutrients. Juicing simply means taking your favorite fruits or vegetables and putting them through a juicing machine. The pulp is taken out, leaving just pure juice, full of minerals and vitamins. My opinion is that your body has to be pretty clean to enjoy God's most beautiful, pure and delicious real food. For the longest time, I would practically become ill if I drank straight vegetable juice. Now that I am less toxic, I really can enjoy juicing and what it offers the body in the way of nutrition. My immune system is much stronger, thanks to the addition of fresh juices to my diet. I enjoy a shot of wheatgrass from time to time, but my favorite juice drink is my own Yoga by Jyl juice. When juicing, make sure your ingredients are all organic.

YOGA BY JYL JUICE

1 handful spinach

1 handful parsley

3 inches cucumber

2 celery stalks

3-4 cloves garlic

2-3 apples

½ lemon

1½ inches fresh ginger root

Ice

For regular juicing, you will, of course, need a juicer. Juicers don't have to be expensive and are a good investment if you are serious about honoring yourself and your health. Starting with the organic greens, the first four ingredients should yield about a ½ cup. Next, add the garlic, apples, lemon and ginger which should yield another ½ cup of juice, so together you will have about 8-10 ounces of freshly squeezed juice. Pour the juice over a glass of ice. In my opinion, the ice is very important. The cool temperature helps to bring out the lemon flavor. I am a Pitta, and if you remember from our earlier discussion about doshas, the Pitta needs cooling down sometimes. It is my truth, but it may also be yours!

Watermelon juice is also a very healthy juice habit. One of my clients gave up her cigarette addiction by drinking watermelon juice. She successfully used watermelon juice to purify and heal her body. She was craving watermelon, because her body knew the effects it would have on her overall health. All she consciously knew was that she felt great. A day didn't go by that she didn't have her juice. I hope we can all feel great and use food to find that healthy and happy feeling.

In terms of its health benefits, watermelon offers the body lycopenes. Lycopenes, carotenoids like beta carotene, deactivate free radicals before they can damage the body's cells. Watermelon and other fruits containing lycopenes may play a role in preventing cancer, heart disease and strokes. So go ahead and spoil yourself, and drink some pretty, pink, cool and sweet juice from a locally grown organic watermelon.

LIVE LONGER SMOOTHIE BY JYL

1 cup kefir

½ cup watermelon juice

½ cup pomegranate or Young Living Ningxia wolfberry juice

1 tablespoon cod liver oil

1 tablespoon Supergreens

2 cups frozen Sambazon acai or frozen blueberries

1. Puree kefir, watermelon juice, pomegranate or wolfberry juice, cod liver oil, Supergreens and frozen berries in a blender until smooth.

2. Garnish the smoothie with your choice of roasted almonds, sunflower seeds, pumpkin seeds, ground flax seeds, wheat germ and a fresh sprig of mint.

Sambazon acai is an excellent replacement for frozen berries. It offers organic essential omegas and is a super antioxidant. Acai is a wild berry harvested by local cooperatives in the Brazilian Amazon. To order call 1-877-726-2276 or go to www.sambazon.com

Describe your current eating and cooking habits.

Notes from Within: _____

How can you start healing with foods?

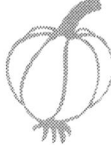

Create Your New Life

First go within and discover what is cooking...

𝒱isualize yourself in perfect health, with great energy all day long, lots of love in your life and being at your ideal body weight. We all deserve to feel good and be the best we can be in life. So many people seek out yoga and meditation to help them feel good and end up creating a whole new lifestyle for themselves. While yoga may have started as a trend (in spite of its long history and practice), it has clearly now been transformed into a lifestyle; a lifestyle that is changing many of us. The body will no longer tolerate unhealthy habits. These old habits will drop off and will be replaced by healthier choices. Grocery stores, restaurants, gyms and retail clothing are changing to keep up with our new needs and demands. Even the yoga studios we have attended will need to change to meet our needs. We will create new sacred places in our world.

Anyone with a life... has stress...
Get balanced and do yoga!

Create a new life by changing the way you think. If you don't like your life, then write a new script. You and you alone have the power to do this. You need to take responsibility for the life you have created, and then move on to the next chapter. Keep your thoughts positive and pure. Happiness begins with dropping the fear in your head and creating love in your heart. Learn to really love yourself by taking the time for a new life cleanse.

A NEW LIFE CLEANSE

Begin gently, and stay in touch with your body and emotions. Have empathy for yourself and let your heart lead the way.

1. Learn to take deep breaths all the way to your belly from time to time during the day.
2. Turn off the TV. I have noticed such clarity in those students who have had the courage to turn off the tube.
3. Try a newspaper break. Our media does a wonderful job at manifesting FEAR and disharmony. As you start feeling calmer and happier, you will naturally want more peace. Let the media scare others not you!
4. Add a lot more water to your diet. Learn to carry a liter with you everywhere you go.
5. Try to eliminate any food addictions in your life.
6. Avoid depending on drugs. I have read that the third leading cause of death in this country is due to prescription drugs.
7. Try to hang out with healthy disciplined people. Birds of a feather flock together. It will make the transition to a healthier you that much easier.
8. Make a list of any and all things you want to change in your life and your diet. Post it in a prominent place where you can see it everyday. Set out to create a new lifestyle.
9. Add more yoga classes to your life. Remember, yoga is a natural cleanse, and it will help you stay focused.
10. At least one day a week, eat only raw fruits and vegetables. Try to notice how your body feels. Notice any emotions that are aroused.
11. Add meditation twice a day… as the sun rises and as the sun sets.
12. Eliminate the drama in your life and stay out of other people's dramas.
13. Write yourself a love letter and read it out loud. What would it mean for you to love yourself?

ONG NAMO GURU DEV NAMO… this mantra, or chant, calls upon the Creator, the Divine Teacher inside every human being.

SELF LOVE TEST...

Find a place where you will not be interrupted for the next 10 minutes. Gently start deepening your breath. Long, deep inhales all the way to your belly, then deep exhales. Feel how the body begins to relax and release tension. Feel how the body quickly and naturally responds to the breath. Now close your eyes and envision a beautiful violet flame in the middle of the room. Allow the flame to grow, filling the room, and see the purifying violet energy enter your body. See the light start at your feet and move up your body. Feel your body release and let go of an old you, to allow a more powerful you to emerge.

Then see in your mind's eye a beautiful golden white light. Allow the light to grow, adding a spiritual essence to your present experience. Let the light enter your body from the top of your head, and flow all the way to your toes. Feel this white golden light heal your body. Now see yourself as the perfect you. You're in perfect health, your body is the perfect weight and size, you have perfect relationships, and you love your work. Notice how you feel. On your next breath, breathe in love and peace, and exhale all negative emotions. Set an intention to be safe, live in harmony and embrace joy. Be grateful to your body, and when you are ready, deepen your breath. Gently stretch your arms over your head, and then open your eyes.

GO WITHIN

Going within has created a new Jyl in the kitchen. Yoga has changed my diet and my consciousness. Meditation, prayer and writing have given me the strength and courage to demand a joy-filled existence and perfect health. It is important that you are aware that this cookbook is my truth. This truth is only my truth at this given time, because tomorrow I may have another truth.

So *Don't believe* me... *Don't believe* this book... *Don't believe* psychics... *Don't believe* your grandfather... *Don't believe* what you read in the paper or watch on TV... *Don't believe* your priest or your doctor... *Don't believe anyone other than your own soul.*

How do you know your soul? Sit and learn to go within. Do believe me when I say that going within can save your life too. Now let's cook up a different you.

I would like to beg you to have patience with everything unresolved in your heart and try to love the questions themselves as if they were locked rooms or books in a very foreign language. Don't search for the answers, which would not be given to you now, because you would not be able to live them. And the point is to live everything.

Live the question now.

--Rainer Maria Rilke

Create your new life. What does it look like?

Can you trust your inner voice? What is it telling you?

Notes from Within: _____

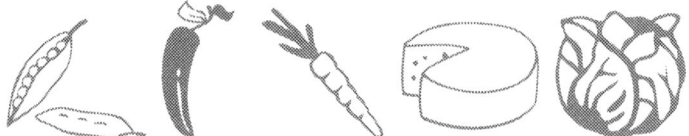

Part Two

FUEL FOR THE JOURNEY

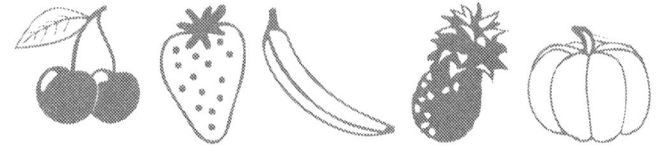

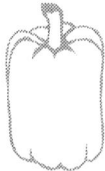

Food to Feed the Soul

I always tell my students, "The only true home you get this lifetime is your body... treat it well and eat for health."

The following recipes are all tried and tested from many of my Yoga and Dinner evenings. Some of the recipes are healthier and better suited for your body than others, so go within and have discernment. Eat, cook and have fun. There is room next to each recipe to add special personal comments. Expect to get 4-6 servings out of each recipe, unless otherwise stated. I give you permission to recreate, add, delete and rock out in your kitchen. Remember to please support your local organic farmers and use only organic foods!

As I mentioned earlier in the book, presentation is everything. How you serve your food is truly influenced by the core of your essence. I encourage all of you to develop your own style in the kitchen. I have been designing my dishes these days by starting with an oversized white porcelain square serving plate. Stacking food is a big trend, so with every dish, I start in the middle of the plate and place a layer of mixed field greens, followed by a favorite grain and finally topped with fish or vegetables. I use garden-grown herbs to crown the dish.

It seems as though the more gourmet the restaurant is, the smaller the portions are. Less is more, and I have to agree. Save room on the plate to use color. Maybe the color comes from a sauce or an edible flower. The presentation should fit your personality. Go ahead and be a little daring with your dishes. Remember, we all eat with our eyes. Presentation should always be a main focus.

Students often ask me -as a longtime yogini- how I eat. Here are my organic food choices in a typical day:

5:30 a.m. one probiotic and a green tea soy latte

7:00 a.m. organic fruit

9:00 a.m. a Live Longer Smoothie by Jyl

11:30 a.m. an organic salad and vegetables with grilled wild salmon

2:00 p.m. a piece of fruit or flaxseed cracker topped with goat cheese

4:00 p.m. a slice of pumpkin almond bread with a green tea latte

8:00 p.m. a piece of fruit, or soup

9:00 p.m. bedtime: probiotic

During the day, I try to drink 3 liters of water.

Supplements: Throughout the day I take supplements, but they will vary. I always make sure I take a probiotic for a healthy colon. I also take a digestive enzyme (especially when I travel), Super Gram Three multiple vitamin, calcium, magnesium and fish oils. Lately, I have been adding Primrose oil to support my hormones and Alpha Lipoic Acid for my liver. Whether you need to add supplements to your diet is strictly up to you. There are many health professionals who can help you determine what is right for your body.

Ocean Foods: Dare to be different and start thinking off the sticky mat. The following might, or might not, be new types of foods for you. Pay attention to ocean foods like dulse, nori, kombu, agar, arame, hijik and wakame. Try adding them to your diet. Let your children try a new healthy treat. I include dulse in my soup stock to add minerals and flavoring. Also try adding these new foods to salads. You will feel how great they are for your health, and you just might start to crave them!

Many of the items I use in my cooking are found at specialty and health food stores. As people become more health conscious, these items are becoming more readily available. Ask your local grocer to stock these items, making them available in your community. There may also be some local stores that currently carry these items, like Jimbo's, Boney's and Henry's in Southern California There are now some national chains catering to a more healthy lifestyle. Stores like Wild Oats, Whole Foods and even Trader Joe's are carrying a wide array of organic and alternative foods.

A reminder: To help you bring doshas into your lifestyle, every recipe will be labeled with symbols. This is helpful when you are feeling out of sorts and need to be balanced. The symbols will identify if the recipe is right for your dosha and offers you the balance you need. Don't worry if your dosha isn't on the dish, you can still enjoy it. Remember, we all have three doshas within us.

Vattas look for the ❀ flower.

Pittas are ☼ sunshine.

Kaphas follow the ❄ snowflake.

Entrees and Side Dishes

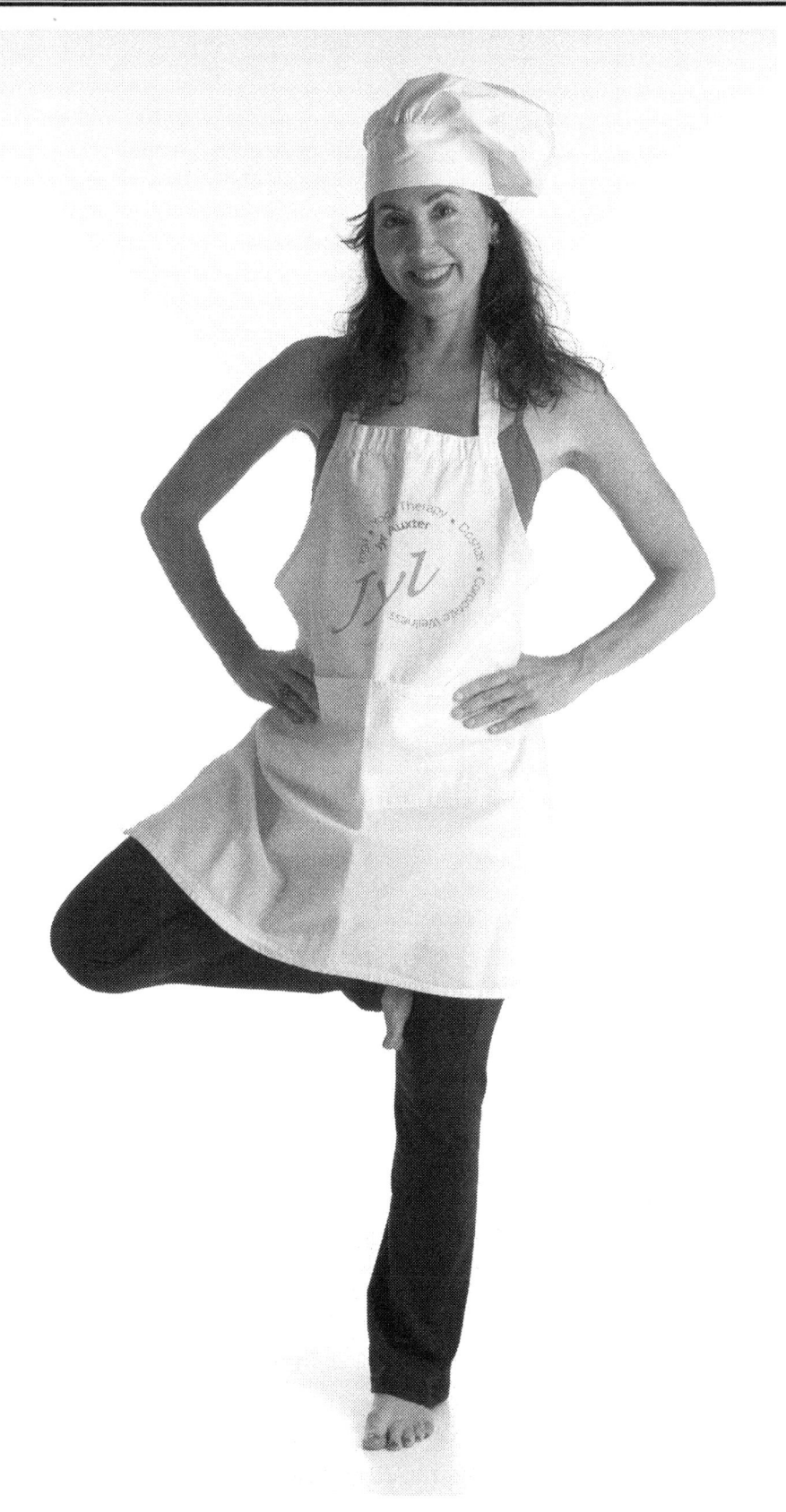

THAI COCONUT CURRIED SALMON WITH GREENS

> Tips: Try replacing the salmon with chicken and top with fresh shredded coconut and granny apples.
>
> If you have fresh ginger leftover, try freezing.

Notes from Within: _____

1 pound wild salmon fillet, skinned
2 tablespoons ghee or butter
1 cup thinly sliced onion
½ teaspoon red curry paste
1-14oz can light coconut milk
2 tablespoons curry powder
1 tablespoon maple syrup
2 tablespoons lime juice
1 tablespoon minced fresh ginger
1 tablespoon fish sauce
2 teaspoons minced garlic
1-8oz bottle clam juice
6 cups watercress or spinach

1. Cook the salmon separately in a medium saucepan. Place enough purified water to cover fish and bring to a boil. Poach the salmon for 10 minutes. The fish will start to have cooked edges. Flip salmon and turn off heat. If you forgot to buy skinned salmon, this is a good time to remove the skin and discard. Let fish continue to cook in saucepan while you are making the curry.

2. In a separate saucepan, heat ghee or butter over medium-high heat, add onions and curry powder. Cook until tender, about 10 minutes.

3. Add coconut milk, curry paste, maple syrup, lime juice, ginger, fish sauce, garlic and clam juice to skillet and continue to cook on low heat.

4. Using your hands, pull salmon apart into bite sized pieces and add to curry. Right before serving, add greens and heat. Serve warm with brown rice or quinoa. Garnish with your favorite lightly sautéed vegetables.

SALMON CAKES

1 pound wild salmon
2 room temperature free-range eggs
1 cup bread crumbs
½ cup Parmesan cheese
½ cup chopped celery
¼ cup chopped scallions
¼ cup chopped fresh dill weed
1 tablespoon celery seed
2 teaspoons cayenne pepper
2 tablespoons ghee or butter

> *Tip: Aged Parmigiano Reggiano is a stimulating cheese choice for your cakes.*

1. In a large bowl, combine salmon, eggs, bread crumbs, Parmesan cheese, celery, scallions, dill, celery seed and cayenne pepper. I really like to use my hands to mix. If the mixture feels too loose, add more bread crumbs.

2. Create patties with mixture.

3. In a frying pan, melt ghee or butter over low heat and add patties. Brown patties on each side (about 5 minutes) and serve on a bed on field greens with a dab of garlic mayonnaise (page 91). Garnish with fresh baby tomatoes, fresh basil and dill weed.

Notes from Within: _____

GARLIC MAYONNAISE

Tip: This mayonnaise tastes great on the salmon cakes and on just about anything you can think of including your finger!

Notes from Within: _____

2 free-range eggs yolks
2 tablespoons raw apple cider vinegar
1 tablespoon fresh lemon juice
¼ teaspoon prepared mustard
¼ teaspoon dill weed
2 cups olive oil
1 teaspoon cayenne pepper
1 teaspoon sea salt
10-15 small cloves garlic
½ fresh garden cucumber, cleaned and peeled

1. In a blender, combine egg yolks, vinegar, lemon juice, mustard, dill and 1 cup oil. Mix into a cream. Add cayenne pepper and sea salt to season.

2. Place whole garlic cloves in a glass pan and drizzle 1 cup olive oil over cloves. In a 350°F oven, bake garlic until golden brown, about 10 minutes.

3. While the garlic is baking, dice cucumber.

4. Let garlic cool, chop and add to mayonnaise along with cucumber. Mix well.

HEALING CRAB CAKES

1 pound real or imitation crab meat
2 room temperature free-range eggs
1 cup bread crumbs
½ cup Parmesan cheese
½ cup chopped celery
¼ cup chopped scallions
¼ cup chopped fresh parsley
2 teaspoons cayenne pepper
2 tablespoons ghee or butter

> Tip: I really like to use imitation crab. I find this white fish to be fabulous for creating crab cakes with a new texture.

1. In a large bowl, combine crab, eggs, bread crumbs, Parmesan cheese, celery, scallions, parsley and pepper. I really like to use my hands to mix. If the mixture feels too loose, add more bread crumbs

2. Create patties with mixture.

3. In a frying pan, melt ghee or butter over low heat and add cakes. Brown cakes on each side (about 5 minutes).

4. Serve cakes on a bed of field greens and rice noodles with raspberry chipotle sauce (page 93) drizzled over the entire dish.

Notes from Within: _____

RASPBERRY CHIPOTLE SAUCE

Tip: Keeps for 7-14 days in refrigerator. Use this sauce with seafood dishes. Perfect with shrimp.

I drizzle the sauce over my Asian Soba Noodle Salad (page 127). These flavors are perfect mates!

2 cups frozen or fresh organic raspberries
¼ cup maple syrup
½ cup chipotle peppers, canned in adobo
2 tablespoons green onions
¼ cup apple cider vinegar
¼ cup white wine or a favorite fruit juice

1. In a saucepan, place raspberries, maple syrup, peppers, green onions, vinegar and wine. Slowly cook for 30 minutes on low heat.

2. Blend in a food processor or blender until smooth.

Notes from Within: _____

_____
_____
_____
_____
_____
_____
_____
_____
_____
_____

SALMON STACK

The dish starts with a circle of raw sprouted hummus (page 94) topped with quinoa tabbouleh (page 95). Poached salmon (page 94) is stacked on top of the tabbouleh. The dish is finished with a pineapple caper salsa (page 96) and pineapple sauce (page 97). Garnish with your favorite greens.

Notes from Within: _____

_____
_____
_____
_____
_____
_____
_____
_____
_____
_____
_____
_____
_____

Poached Salmon

1 pound wild salmon, skinned
1-16oz can coconut milk

1. Place salmon in a large saucepan with coconut milk over medium heat. Make sure the fish is covered. You may have to add some purified water. Poach for 10 minutes on each side.

Raw Sprouted Hummus

2 cups sprouted chickpeas (garbanzo beans) (sprouting time 2 days, page 70)
½ cup chopped fresh parsley
¼ cup freshly squeezed lemon juice
1 tablespoon minced garlic
¼ cup tahini
¼ cup olive oil
2 teaspoons ground allspice
1 teaspoon sea salt

1. Place the chickpeas in a covered glass jar with purified water until the grain is covered and soak for eight hours. After soaking the chickpeas, drain and place in a colander and continue to rinse daily. The chickpeas will to sprout within two days. After grain has sprouted, refrigerate.

2. Drain and rinse sprouted chickpeas. In a blender, combine chickpeas with parsley, lemon juice, garlic, tahini, olive oil, allspice and sea salt. Blend until smooth.

SALMON STACK

> Tip: Quinoa is rich in protein, potassium and phosphorus. It is a perfect replacement for rice or wheat.

Notes from Within: _____

Sprouted Quinoa Tabbouleh

¼ cup sprouted quinoa (page 70)
1 ½ cup diced ripe tomatoes
2 teaspoons sea salt
¼ cup freshly squeezed lemon juice
½ cup chopped fresh mint
¼ cup chopped scallions
¼ cup diced cucumber
1 ½ cup chopped fresh parsley
3-5 cloves garlic, crushed
1 teaspoon minced fresh ginger
½ cup olive oil
cayenne pepper to taste

1. To sprout, place quinoa in a glass container filled with purified water. Soak grain for two hours, covered. The glass container can sit out on kitchen counter. Drain quinoa using a colander. Leave the grain in the colander and for 2 days rinse with water. After a couple of days the grain will start to sprout. Sprouts keep 3 days in refrigerator.

2. In a large mixing bowl, combine sprouted quinoa, tomatoes, sea salt, lemon juice, mint, scallions, cucumber, parsley, garlic, ginger, olive oil and cayenne pepper. Toss to mix.

Pineapple Caper Pepper Salsa

1 fresh ripe pineapple, chopped
2 vine ripe tomatoes, diced
1 small red onion, diced
½ cup diced apples
½ cup halved green grapes
½ cup diced cucumber
2 cups freshly squeezed lemon juice
½ cup capers
Freshly ground black pepper to taste

1. Chop pineapple, tomatoes, onion, apples, grapes and cucumber. Place in a large bowl.
2. Cover with lemon juice.
3. Add capers and pepper.
4. Chill and serve.

SALMON STACK

Tip: Sometimes I will add watermelon juice, or pineapple juice to the mixture to add sweetness.

Notes from Within: _____

SALMON STACK

Tip: When I serve the salmon stack dish I splash the pineapple sauce around the edges of the plate. It really adds a gourmet presentation.

Notes from Within: _____

Pineapple sauce

2 cups concentrated pineapple juice
1 cup soy sauce
¼ cup maple syrup
½ cup crushed fresh or frozen pineapple
2 cloves garlic, crushed
2 tablespoons strawberry jelly
1 tablespoon chopped fresh ginger
1 tablespoon sesame oil
½ teaspoon raw apple cider vinegar
Black pepper to taste

1. In a saucepan, combine juice, soy sauce, maple syrup, pineapple, garlic, jelly, ginger, sesame oil, vinegar and pepper. Bring to a boil.

2. Reduce heat and cook for 40 minutes on low heat to thicken sauce.

PISTACHIO-SALMON

1 pound fresh wild salmon
2 tablespoons apple juice
2 tablespoons soy sauce
1 tablespoon grated fresh ginger
2 tablespoons sesame oil
2 tablespoons chopped pistachio nuts

1. Combine apple juice, soy sauce, ginger and sesame oil. Add salmon and marinate overnight in a large bowl.

2. When ready to cook, place salmon in a large saucepan and cook 3-5 minutes on each side. Garnish with pistachio nuts and serve on a bed of fresh spinach leaves.

Notes from Within: _____
_____
_____
_____
_____
_____
_____
_____
_____
_____
_____
_____
_____
_____
_____
_____
_____
_____

PAN-FRIED SCALLOPS WITH TRUFFLE AND GRAPE SAUCE

Notes from Within: _____

_____
_____
_____
_____
_____
_____
_____
_____
_____
_____
_____
_____

Truffle Sauce:

1 yellow onion, chopped
2 tablespoons ghee or butter
1 carrot, peeled and chopped
1 ½ cups chicken broth
1 ½ cups wine or purified water
1 tablespoon truffle juice

1. In a sauce pan, sauté onion in ghee or butter until tender.
2. Add carrots, broth, wine and truffle juice. Bring to a boil, reduce heat and simmer for 20 minutes.

Grape Sauce:

1 tablespoon ghee or butter
2 tablespoons chicken broth
¼ pound red grapes

1. In a saucepan, melt ghee or butter and add chicken broth. Stir in grapes. Let cook for 30 minutes
2. Puree grape sauce in blender.

Scallops:

10 large scallops
2 tablespoons ghee or butter
¼ cup white wine

1. In a saucepan, sauté scallops in ghee or butter, then add wine. Simmer scallops in wine for 10 minutes until cooked.
2. Place scallops on plate. Top with truffle and grape sauce.

SHRIMP AND SCALLOP KABOBS

1 cup olive oil
6 cloves garlic, crushed
2 cups freshly squeezed lemon juice
4 tablespoons chopped fresh parsley
1 stalk lemongrass, thinly sliced
2 tablespoons chopped fresh ginger
1 cup dry white wine
1 pound shrimp and scallops, cleaned

1. Combine olive oil, garlic, lemon juice, parsley, lemongrass and white wine to create a marinade.

2. Add seafood. Marinate overnight or at least 4 hours.

3. Place fish on skewer and grill. Fish will cook fast, about 3 minutes on each side. Do not over cook!

Notes from Within: _____

SHELLFISH RISOTTO

> Tip: While cooking the clams and mussels, shake the pan occasionally... wake up those little guys. If not the shells may not open.

Notes from Within: _____

_____
_____
_____
_____
_____
_____
_____
_____
_____
_____
_____
_____
_____

2 ¼ cups fish stock
1 ½ cups Arborio rice
1 pound clams, cleaned
1 ½ pounds mussels, cleaned
2 tablespoons olive oil
4 cloves garlic, crushed
2 ounces medium shrimp, cleaned
6 ounces squid, cut into thin rings
1 cup chopped fresh parsley
1 cup dry white wine
4 tablespoons ghee or butter
cayenne pepper and sea salt to taste

1. Bring fish stock to a boil, add rice and cook for 20 minutes. Reduce heat and cover for 10 more minutes.
2. In a separate pan, cook clams in ¼ cup of water. Cover and cook until clams open. Cook mussels in the same fashion. Shake pan while cooking to open clams and mussels.
3. In a large frying pan, brown garlic in oil.
4. Add shrimp and squid to garlic. Cook for 3 minutes.
5. Add rice, shellfish, parsley, wine, ghee or butter, cayenne pepper and sea salt to shrimp and squid. Garnish with fresh watercress.

DOSHA PASTA DISH

Pasta:

2 cups spelt flour
1 cup fava flour
2 teaspoons cayenne pepper
1 teaspoon sea salt
3 eggs
¼ cup chopped fresh dill weed
1 teaspoon olive oil
2 quarts purified water

1. In a mixing bowl, sift flours, cayenne papper and sea salt together and mix. Place mixture on a flat floured surface.

2. Create a well in the middle of the flour. Add eggs, dill weed and oil.

3. Use hands to mix. Knead pasta flour until smooth. Set aside and cover with plastic. Let dough rest for an hour.

4. Roll out dough and use knife or pasta machine to cut pasta.

5. Boil water. Drop pasta in water and when the pasta surfaces (2-3 minutes) it is done. Don't over cook.

> Tip: When you use flours like spelt and fava, you are creating a flavorful, healthy, high protein pasta. My students didn't even know they were eating pasta!!

Notes from Within: _____

DOSHA PASTA DISH

Notes from Within: _____

Topping:

2 tablespoons olive oil
3 cloves garlic, crushed
¼ cup whole pine nuts
1 cup chopped peeled carrots
2 cups chopped tomatoes
1 cup sliced daikon
½ cup chopped shiitake mushrooms
1 cup fresh green peas
½ cup sliced red peppers

1. In a wok, brown garlic and pine nuts in olive oil. Add carrots, tomatoes, daikon, mushrooms, peas and red peppers and stir-fry. Add more oil and a little Aged Parmigiano Reggiano if desired.

2. Serve over pasta.

BEET GREENS AND GOAT CHEESE RAVIOLI

Dosha pasta (page 102), rolled into 4 sheets
2 bunches baby beets and greens, chopped
1 tablespoon ghee or butter
6 cloves garlic, crushed
½ cup goat cheese
1 tablespoon nutmeg
½ teaspoon cayenne pepper
½ teaspoon sea salt
2 tablespoons chopped fresh marjoram
¼ cup freshly grated Parmesan cheese
½ cup white wine
½ cup olive oil
2 tablespoons chopped fresh sage

> Tip: When you are cooking beets remember to cut off greens and roots. Simply place the whole beet into the water (no need to peel). Make sure the water is covering each beet and simmer for one hour. When tender, place into cold water. You can use your hands to rub off skin to clean. Very easy!

1. Make dosha pasta the day before and refrigerate. Also the day before, cook beets (save greens) for an hour under low heat and rinse with cool water. Clean and chop the beets and greens. Refrigerate.

2. In a saucepan, sauté garlic in ghee or butter. Add beet greens, goat cheese, nutmeg, cayenne pepper, sea salt, marjoram and Parmesan cheese to saucepan and cook over medium heat for 5 minutes.

3. Place pasta on a flat surface. Use a 2 ½ inch round cookie cutter to cut six circles from each sheet.

4. Spoon in 1 teaspoon of beet filling. Lightly brush edges with water and fold over into a semicircle shape.

5. Bring a large pot of water to a boil and cook pasta for 5 minutes.

6. Drain and place pasta into a saucepan. Lightly brown ravioli in olive oil. Add wine and sage, and serve with chopped cooked beets

Notes from Within: _____

LINGUINE WITH CHARD AND PINE NUTS

Notes from Within: _____

1 pound pasta
1 bunch chard, chopped
2 medium vine ripened tomatoes, chopped
1 medium onion, chopped
½ cup chopped fresh basil
2 tablespoons chopped fresh parsley
¼ cup chopped black olives (optional)
⅓ cup olive oil
6 large cloves garlic, crushed
¼ cup whole pine nuts
1 tablespoon freshly ground pepper
optional: grated Parmesan cheese

1. Buy or make Dosha Pasta (page 102). Cook and have ready.

2. Chop chard, tomatoes, onion, basil, parsley and olives.

3. In a large saucepan, add oil, garlic, pine nuts and sauté. Add chopped vegetables and lightly cook.

4. Toss pasta into vegetable mixture. Season with pepper and top with cheese.

MUSTARD CHICKEN WITH THYME

2 cups Italian bread crumbs
¼ cup chopped fresh thyme
¼ cup chopped fresh rosemary
1 cup freshly grated Parmesan cheese
sea salt and pepper to taste
2 tablespoons olive oil
6 free-range chicken breasts
6 tablespoons honey mustard
1 ½ cups white wine

> *Tip: This is a very easy and fast dinner.*

1. In a bowl, combine bread crumbs, thyme, rosemary, cheese and seasonings. Set aside.

2. Drizzle 1 tablespoon of oil in bottom of baking pan and place chicken breasts in pan.

3. Spread mustard on top of each breast. Sprinkle bread crumb mixture to cover chicken. Drizzle rest of olive oil on top of chicken and place wine in bottom of baking pan. Bake covered for 30 minutes at 350° F.

4. Serve with brown rice and steamed vegetables. A great garnish for this chicken dish is chopped mint leaves and field ripe tomatoes.

Notes from Within: _____

THAI CHICKEN WITH PEANUTS

> Tip: I sometimes add freshly grounded peanut butter to this dish if I am craving a more peanut flavor.
>
> Most grocery stores will carry fish sauce and curry paste in their Asian section. Ask your local grocer.

Notes from Within: _____

_____
_____
_____
_____
_____
_____
_____
_____
_____
_____

2 tablespoons fish sauce
2 tablespoons freshly squeezed lime juice
2 tablespoons maple syrup
1 teaspoon red curry paste
¼ cup purified water
2 tablespoons olive oil
1 pound free-range chicken breast, boneless and skinless
½ cup minced shallots
1 stalk lemongrass, thinly sliced
1 tablespoon chopped fresh ginger
½ cup chopped Asian basil leaves
½ cup chopped peanuts

1. In a bowl, combine fish sauce, lime juice, syrup, curry paste and ¼ cup water (may use wine or juice instead of water).

2. Heat oil in a large skillet over medium-high heat. Add chicken, shallots, lemongrass and ginger, sauté for 5-7 minutes, or until chicken is cooked.

3. Add fish-sauce mixture and cook 3 minutes. Stir in fresh basil. Spoon onto platter over brown rice, top with peanuts.

FREE-RANGE CHICKEN AND BUCKWHEAT SOBA DISH

2 free-range chicken breasts
1 teaspoon sea salt
2 tablespoons olive oil
½ cup white wine
1 package buckwheat soba noodles
1 cup peanut sauce (page 109)
1 cup grated peeled carrots
6 green onions, thinly sliced
½ cup chopped fresh cilantro
1 cup daikon radish sprouts
1 cup sprouted sunflower seeds
2 tablespoons soy sauce
1 tablespoon flaxseed oil
1 teaspoon cayenne pepper

> *Tip: A great dish to use the peanut sauce.*

1. *To prepare chicken:* Set oven to 375°F. Rub chicken with sea salt and olive oil. Place in pan, add ½ cup white wine. Roast chicken covered for 30 minutes.

2. *To prepare noodles:* Place soba noodles in boiling water for 3-5 minutes to cook. Do not over cook noodles.

3. In a mixing bowl, combine peanut sauce, noodles and bites size chunks of roasted chicken. Add carrots, green onions, cilantro and sprouts.

4. Toss mixture and add soy sauce, flaxseed oil and cayenne pepper.

Notes from Within: _____

PEANUT SAUCE

6 cloves garlic, crushed
4 green onions, chopped
½ cup chopped fresh cilantro
½ cup freshly ground peanut butter
¼ cup tamari or soy sauce
2 tablespoons freshly squeezed lemon juice
½ cup purified water
1 tablespoon chopped fresh ginger

1. In a blender or food processor combine garlic, green onions, cilantro, peanut butter, tamari, lemon juice, water and ginger.
2. Blend until smooth.

Tip: If the mixture becomes too thick, add water to change consistency. The peanut sauce is easier to work with if it is on the runny saucy side.

For a healthy peanut butter, I go to a health food store and grind my own peanut butter, right in the store!

Notes from Within: _____

GRILLED CHICKEN SKEWERS

4 free-range chicken breasts, boneless and skinless
1 bottle dark beer
6 cloves garlic, crushed
2 tablespoons freshly squeezed lemon juice
2 tablespoons chopped fresh rosemary
4 tablespoons soy sauce

1. Marinate chicken in beer, garlic, lemon juice, rosemary and soy sauce for 4 hours in refrigerator.

2. Chop chicken into 2 inch pieces and place on metal skewers.

3. On a heated grill, cook chicken for about 15 minutes on each side.

4. Serve chicken with fresh summer mango salsa (page 111) for an appetizer.

Notes from Within: _____

SUMMER MANGO SALSA

1 large ripe mango, diced
1 cup chopped fresh pineapple
1 vine ripe tomato, chopped
¼ cup diced scallions
¼ cup chopped fresh cilantro
2 tablespoons freshly squeezed lime juice

1. In a large mixing bowl combine mango, pineapple, tomato, scallions, cilantro and cover with lime juice.
2. Refrigerate and keep up to two days.

> Tip: Mangos have a large flat seed, so cut it lengthwise on both sides of the seed. Then score the fruit, turn the skin inside out, and cut off your diced mango!

Notes from Within: _____

TURKEY CAROB MOLE WITH ALMONDS AND SESAME SEEDS

Roast Turkey Breasts

6 breasts free-range turkey

4 cloves garlic, crushed

1 teaspoon sea salt

4 tablespoons (½ stick) organic butter

½ cup organic free-range chicken stock

¼ cup fresh lemon juice

1. Set oven to 375° F. Rub the turkey with garlic, salt and butter. Place turkey in a roasting pan, add chicken stock and lemon juice. Roast for 30 minutes. Let turkey cool, then slice.

2. Prepare mole (page 113).

Tip: Mole is traditionally made with chocolate. Carob is a lovely substitute and not as hard on the digestive system.

This is a great new Thanksgiving feast!

Notes from Within: _____

TURKEY CAROB MOLE WITH ALMONDS AND SESAME SEEDS

Tip: Please pay attention when handling the chiles. Do not rub your eyes or put your hand to your mouth. Wash your hands carefully.

Notes from Within: _____

_____
_____
_____
_____
_____
_____
_____
_____
_____
_____

Mole with Almonds and Sesame Seeds

¼ Mulato chile, diced

3 Pasillas chiles, diced

3 Anchos chiles, diced

¼ cup chopped soaked almonds (page 70)

¼ cup chopped peanuts

2 tablespoons olive oil

¼ cup raw sesame seeds

1 teaspoon chile seeds

5 cloves garlic, crushed

1 cup turkey stock

½ onion, chopped

1 cup white wine

4 squares carob

1 tablespoon ground anise

1 tablespoon ground cloves

2 tablespoons ground cinnamon

1 teaspoon cayenne pepper

1 tablespoon maple syrup

1. Dice chiles and nuts.

2. In a saucepan, add olive oil and sauté sesame and chile seeds, garlic, chiles and nuts for about 5 minutes.

3. Add turkey stock, onion, wine, carob, anise, cloves, cinnamon, cayenne pepper and maple syrup. Cook for 30 minutes.

4. Serve this savory sauce with roasted free-range turkey breast (page 112) and garlic mashed potatoes. Surround the dish with fresh steamed English peas and fresh cranberries. Drizzle your beautiful mole sauce over the whole plate.

SAFFRON RICE

3 cups basmati rice

5 cups water

4 tablespoons ghee or butter

¼ cup whole pine nuts

1 ½ cups fresh peas

½ cup white wine or chicken stock

1 tablespoon ground saffron

1 tablespoon honey

4 tablespoons olive oil

1 teaspoon sea salt

1 tablespoon soy sauce

1. Place rice and water in a rice cooker or saucepan. Cover and simmer for 20 minutes or until done.

2. In another saucepan, melt ghee or butter and add pine nuts. Lightly brown pine nuts.

3. Add peas, wine or stock, honey and saffron to pine nuts. Cook for 5 minutes or until peas have softened.

4. Finally, add cooked rice and oil to mixture. Season to taste with sea salt and soy sauce.

Notes from Within: _____

GRILLED VEGETABLES

Notes from Within: _____

Marinade:

1 cup olive oil
¼ cup apple cider vinegar
10 medium size cloves garlic, crushed
1 ½ cups chopped fresh basil leaves
¼ cup chopped fresh rosemary
1 cup freshly squeezed lemon juice
1 cup white wine
1 teaspoon sea salt
Freshly grounded pepper to taste

Vegetables to Grill:

3 carrots, peeled
2 zucchinis
1 eggplant
2 summer squash
2 red peppers
2 leeks
2 Portobella mushrooms

1. Clean and creatively slice vegetables.
2. Combine olive oil, vinegar, garlic, basil, rosemary, lemon juice, wine, sea salt and pepper in a large bowl. Add vegetables and marinate for 3 hours in refrigerator.
3. Grill vegetables for about five minutes on each side.
4. Serve with brown rice or on a bed of greens if you are watching calories.

SPINACH AND ASPARAGUS

2 tablespoons olive oil

3 cloves garlic, crushed

8 asparagus stalks, cleaned (break the stalk and discard the bottom)

1 teaspoon cayenne pepper

2 cups fresh spinach leaves

2 tablespoons goat cheese

1. Heat oil in saucepan and add garlic, asparagus tips and cayenne pepper. Cook on medium heat for about 5 minutes.

2. Add spinach and cook just a minute more or until spinach starts to wilt.

3. Top dish with goat cheese.

> Tip: I use chavrie goat cheese with basil and roasted garlic.

Notes from Within: _____

CARROTS, ASPARAGUS AND TARRAGON

Tip: The tarragon leaf can be separated from the stalk very easily by running your fingers up the stalk.

Notes from Within: _____

2 tablespoons ghee or butter

1 pound carrots, peeled

1 pound fresh asparagus, cleaned (break the stalk and discard the bottom)

3 tablespoons honey

¼ cup white wine or orange juice

3 tablespoons fresh tarragon leaves (see tip)

sea salt and pepper to taste

1. Clean and cut the carrots and asparagus into long wedges.

2. Heat ghee or butter in saucepan. Add carrots and asparagus. Lightly cook for 5-10 minutes.

3. Add honey, wine or juice and tarragon. Let dish sit while you prepare the rest of the meal.

4. Serve as a side dish, or on a bed of spinach for a main course. Season with sea salt and freshly ground pepper.

WATERMELON MASHED CARROTS

1 pound carrots, peeled, cleaned and chopped
½ cup fresh watermelon juice
¼ cup whipping cream
2 tablespoons maple syrup
1 tablespoon soy sauce

1. In a pot, boil 2 quarts of water and add chopped carrots. Cook carrots for 20 minutes over low to medium heat.

2. Drain carrots and place in blender or food processor.

3. Add juice, cream and maple syrup and blend until creamy. Add soy sauce to taste.

> *Tip: This is a perfect substitute for mashed potatoes. The carrots are the most beautiful red color and really add to the appearance of a plate.*

Notes from Within: _____

_____
_____
_____
_____
_____
_____
_____
_____
_____
_____
_____

PUMPKIN AND VEGETABLE TOFU STIR-FRY

Notes from Within: _____
_____
_____
_____
_____
_____
_____
_____
_____
_____
_____
_____
_____
_____
_____
_____
_____

1 small raw pumpkin, diced
1 small head broccoli, chopped
1 cup fresh or frozen sweet green peas
1 bundle raw kale, chopped
1 package herb tofu, chopped
2 tablespoons unrefined coconut oil
3 cloves garlic, crushed
1 teaspoon ground cinnamon
1 teaspoon ground nutmeg
1 teaspoon ground cloves
sea salt to taste

1. Clean and chop pumpkin, broccoli and kale. Cut tofu into small cubes.

2. In a large wok, heat oil and brown garlic. Add tofu and lightly brown. Push tofu to the side and add more oil to wok if needed.

3. Add pumpkin, broccoli, peas and kale and lightly cook. Toss tofu, vegetables, cinnamon, nutmeg and cloves together in wok and serve on brown rice. Salt to taste.

PRAYER BEANS

Tip: I call these Prayer Beans because after you eat them, you will feel blessed!

4 slices turkey bacon (optional)
2 yellow onions, chopped
½ cup chopped green bell pepper
½ cup chopped red bell pepper
4 cloves garlic, crushed
2 cups chopped tomatoes
½ cup purified water
¼ cup dark molasses
¼ cup maple syrup
2 tablespoons apple cider vinegar
1 tablespoon Bragg Liquid Aminos
2 tablespoons chopped fresh basil
2 teaspoons dry mustard
½ teaspoon sea salt
¼ teaspoon cayenne pepper
3 cups cooked cannellini or northern beans
3 cups black beans
Optional: add a variety of beans or maybe use only one type if they are your favorite.

1. In a soup pot, cook bacon until crispy. Drain and save drippings. Chop and set bacon aside.

2. In a frying pan, heat 2 tablespoons of drippings and add onion, bell peppers and garlic. Saute until tender.

3. Stir in tomatoes, water, molasses, syrup, vinegar, Braggs, basil, mustard, sea salt and cayenne pepper.

4. Stir in beans and bacon. Heat for 20 minutes.

Notes from Within: _____

BRAISED BABY BOK CHOY

❄

4 tablespoons ghee or butter
½ cup chopped walnuts
1 teaspoon vanilla
1 pound baby bok choy, trimmed and cleaned
½ cup chicken stock
1 tablespoon hot sesame oil

Notes from Within: _____

1. In a large saucepan, place 1 tablespoon ghee or butter, walnuts and vanilla. Brown the walnuts and set aside.

2. Place the remaining ghee or butter in saucepan. Add bok choy and lightly brown. Add chicken stock and cook another 2 minutes.

3. Serve bok choy on a bed of rice. Pour stock over dish and add hot oil.

4. Top this healthy meal off with walnuts.

ACORN SQUASH WITH MILLET

2 medium size acorn squash
2 tablespoons ghee or butter
½ cup millet
1 cup purified water
2 tablespoons maple syrup
1 tablespoon vanilla
2 tablespoons chopped walnuts

1. Wash off squash and cut in half. Preheat oven to 350°F. Place squash face down on non-stick cookie sheet. Bake for 30 minutes.

2. In a saucepan, place one tablespoon ghee or butter and millet. Brown millet in ghee or butter. Add one cup purified water to millet. Cover and cook for 20 minutes, allowing water to cook off.

3. Combine millet with maple syrup, vanilla and walnuts.

4. Flip squash and stuff with millet mixture. Bake for another 20 minutes.

5. Drizzle dish with maple syrup

> *Tip: I also like to add dried black currents and fresh cooked vegetables to the millet. Now it becomes a whole meal.*
>
> *Millet is a perfect grain for your health because it is alkaline.*

Notes from Within: _____

MILLET CAKES

Tip: If you eat fish, you might add the fish on top of the cakes. Finish the dish with your favorite chutney and a tangerine sauce.

Notes from Within: _____

4 tablespoons unrefined coconut oil
2 cups millet
1 cup purified water
¼ cup chopped fresh kale
¼ cup chopped broccoli
1 tablespoon chopped green onions
2 tablespoons chopped fresh dill weed
½ orange bell pepper, chopped
½ cup mashed soft tofu
1 teaspoon cayenne pepper
Optional: grated favorite cheese

1. In a saucepan, heat 1 tablespoon oil. Add millet and lightly brown. Add water, cover and cook for 20 minutes, allowing water to cook off.

2. In another saucepan, lightly sauté kale, broccoli, green onions, dill and bell pepper in 1 tablespoon coconut oil while millet is cooking.

3. In a large bowl, combine tofu, cayenne pepper, vegetables, cooled millet and cheese. Make patties and transfer back to saucepan. Lightly brown in remaining oil.

4. On a plate, add favorite field greens. Top the greens with the millet cakes.

PEA PANCAKES

1 cup fresh or frozen peas
2 tablespoons soy milk
1 tablespoon cream
1 free-range egg
¼ cup fava flour
1 tablespoon maple syrup
¼ teaspoon sea salt
½ teaspoon baking powder
4 tablespoons ghee or butter

Tip: For a complete meal, serve with lightly sautéd julianned fresh vegetables.

1. Cook fresh peas or let frozen peas thaw. In blender or food processor, add milk, cream and peas. Puree.

2. Add egg, flour, maple syrup, sea salt, baking powder and ghee or butter to blender. Blend mixture until smooth. Add more liquid if necessary.

3. Cook like you would any pancake. Garnish with scallions, plain yogurt and fresh tomatoes.

Notes from Within: _____

Salads

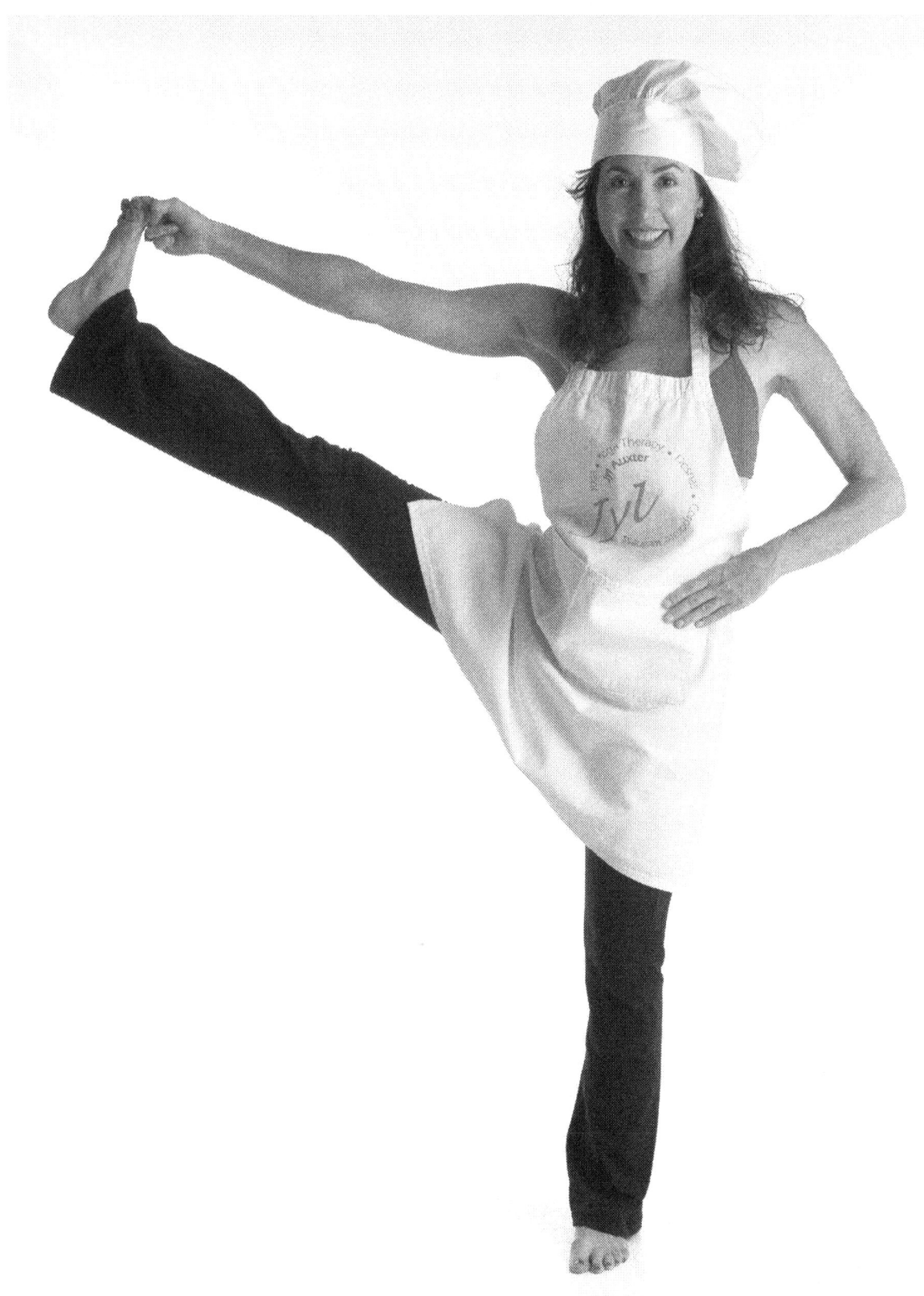

ASIAN NOODLE SALAD WITH TOASTED SESAME DRESSING

Salad:

1-8oz package buckwheat soba noodles
¼ cup toasted sesame seeds
¼ cup chopped cilantro leaves
½ cup chopped scallions
¼ cup chopped red cabbage

Dressing:

3 tablespoons toasted sesame oil
4 tablespoons tamari or soy sauce
4 tablespoons balsamic vinegar
1 tablespoon maple syrup
1 tablespoon hot pepper oil

1. Cook soba noodles for 3-5 minutes. Make sure not to over cook.
2. Combine noodles with sesame seeds and chopped cilantro, scallions and cabbage. Toss in dressing.
3. Garnish with additional toasted sesame seeds and cilantro.

Tip: Some people will not eat pasta because it is the "F" word... fattening... oops. I said it. Remind your guests that this dish has 359 calories per serving, 16 grams at, 40% fat calories, 0 mg. cholesterol, 44 grams carbohydrates, and 11 grams protein.

These noodles offer a great healthy meal to your body.

Notes from Within: _____

ARUGULA AND KALE SALAD

4 tablespoons olive oil
1 teaspoon prepared mustard
1 tablespoon freshly squeezed lemon juice
1-2 bunches fresh arugula, chopped
1-2 bunches fresh kale, chopped
1 medium cucumber, chopped
1 carrot, chopped
1 red bell pepper, chopped
¼ cup chopped walnuts
Optional: 3 tablespoons Parmesan cheese

> Tip: Chopped fresh mint leaves add a lot of flavor to this salad.

1. In a large bowl, mix olive oil, mustard and lemon juice for dressing.
2. Toss arugula, kale, cucmber, carrot and bell pepper with salad dressing. Add walnuts and season to taste.
3. Serve on chilled salad plates.

Notes from Within: _____

HEALTHY RAW SALAD

❄

Tip: Use any sprouts that you like. If you are not familiar with sprouts go to the health food store and check them out. Remember you can make your own sprouts.

1 cup sprouted aduki beans
1 cup sprouted lentils
1 cup sprouted mung beans
1 cup sunflower sprouts
4 stalks celery, chopped
3 red bell peppers, chopped
1 cup chopped leeks
2 ears fresh corn, off the cob
4 cloves garlic, crushed
1 cup freshly squeezed lemon juice
1 tablespoon Bragg Liquid Aminos
2 tablespoons olive oil
1 tablespoon ground cumin
1 tablespoon chili powder

Notes from Within: _____

1. Combine sprouts in a big salad bowl.
2. Prepare celery, bell peppers and leeks by chopping and adding them to sprouts.
3. Corn is placed in pan of 2 quarts boiling water. Let cook for 2 minutes and turn off heat. Keep corn in water for 5 minutes while you prepare the dressing. Drain corn and let cool.
4. In a seperate bowl, mix garlic, lemon juice, Bragg Aminos and olive oil. Sprinkle in cumin and chili powder.
5. Cut corn off cob. Add corn and dressing to salad bowl. Toss. Let marinate for two hours in refrigerator.

BEET SALAD WITH TOASTED PUMPKIN SEEDS

4 large red beets
2 quarts water or enough to cover beets
2 tablespoons melted ghee or butter
¼ cup pumpkin seeds
2 cups olive oil
2 tablespoons apple cider vinegar
2 scallions, chopped
1 tablespoon maple syrup
¼ pound feta cheese, crumbled
1 bunch beet greens, chopped

1. Place beets and water in a medium size sauce pan and cook over high heat until the water starts to boil. Lower heat and simmer for an hour.

2. While beets are cooking, coat pumpkin seeds with ghee or butter and spread on cookie sheet Bake at 350°F for 30 minutes.

3. Cook beets until tender. Using a colander, drain beets and rinse with cold water. Peel, clean, and slice beets.

4. Combine olive oil, vinegar, scallions, syrup, beets and cheese. Toss ingredients.

5. Place beets on greens. Top with toasted pumpkin seeds.

Tip: When cooking and cleaning beets, be careful of the red beet juice. It will stain your towels, hands and clothes.

Notes from Within: _____

PORTABELLA & SHIITAKE MUSHROOMS ON ARUGULA SALAD

5 ounces arugula, chopped
2 tablespoons olive oil
1 tablespoon Balsamic vinegar
½ tablespoon maple syrup
1 tablespoon Dijon-style mustard
4 large Portabella mushrooms, brush to clean
7-10 small Shiitake mushrooms, brush to clean
4 tablespoons crumbled goat cheese
2 fresh ripe pears, sliced

1. Clean and chop arugula. Set aside in refrigerator.
2. Mix olive oil, vinegar, maple syrup and mustard.
3. Brush mushrooms with extra olive oil and place under broiler or on a heated grill. Broil for 5-6 minutes on each side.
4. Have four chilled salad plates available. When you are ready to serve, toss greens with dressing and top with mushrooms, cheese and pears.

> *Tip: If I have a ripe avocado, I like to add it along with any fresh herbs... basil or mint are wonderful additions.*
>
> *Cleaning Mushrooms: There is actually a small brush made to clean mushroons. If you don't have one, use a paper towel. Avoid using water to clean mushrooms.*

Notes from Within: _____

Soups

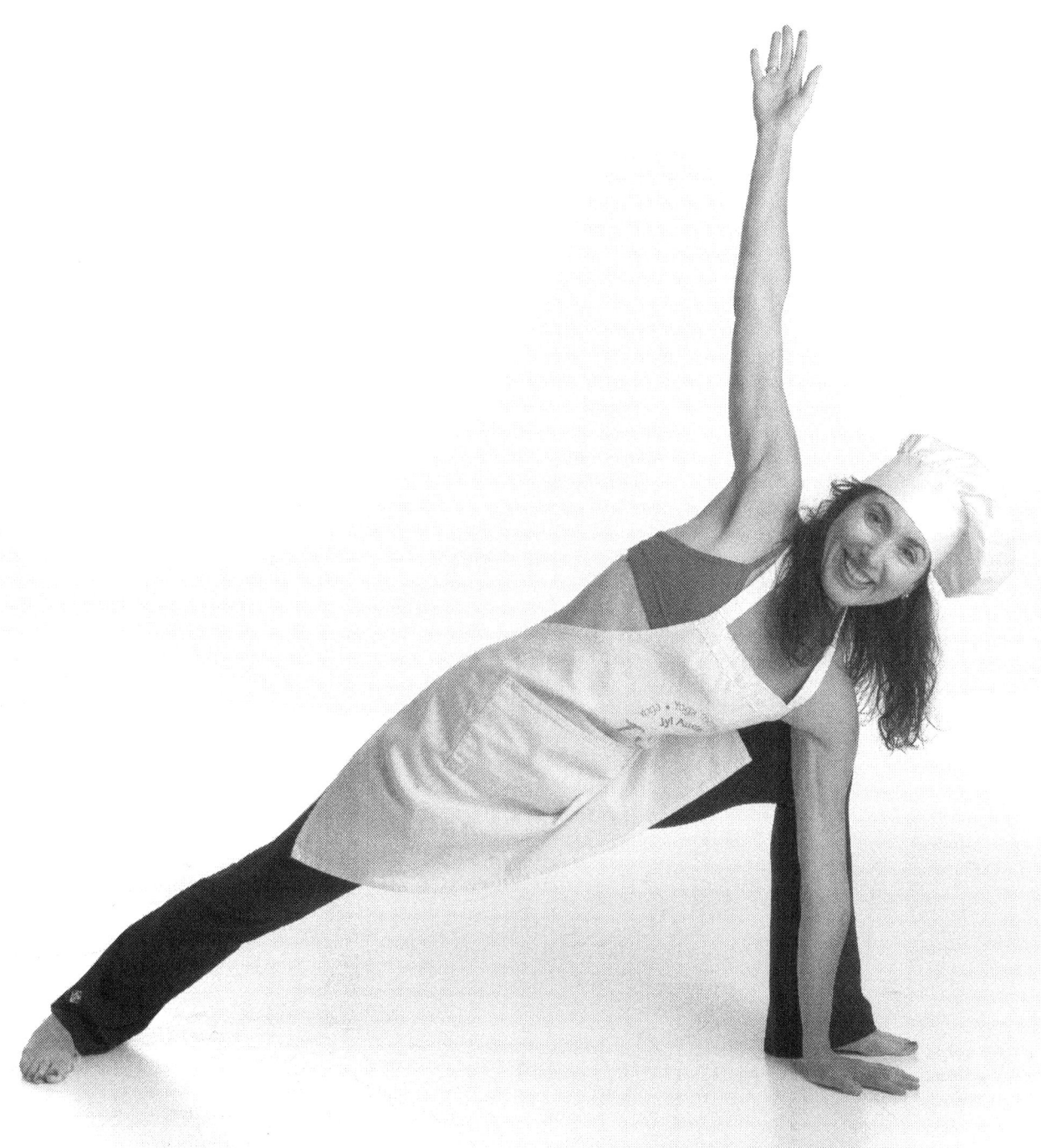

PUMPKIN SOUP

> Tip: EXTRA easy soup to prepare!!!! I love this soup in the winter and it is perfect for the holidays.

Notes from Within: _____

¼ cup ghee or butter
1 cup chopped onion
6 cloves garlic, crushed
2 teaspoons curry powder
1 teaspoon sea salt
2 teaspoons ground coriander
2 teaspoons crushed red pepper
3 cups chicken broth
1 ¾ cups (16 ounces) pumpkin pie filling
1 cup soy milk or whipping cream
1 tablespoon plain yogurt
½ cup chopped fresh chives

1. In a large saucepan, melt butter and sauté onion and garlic for 5 minutes.
2. Add curry powder, sea salt, coriander and red pepper to the saucepan and cook for 2 minutes.
3. Add broth, bring to a boil, reduce heat and simmer uncovered for 15 minutes.
4. Stir in pumpkin and cream or soy milk and continue to cook over low heat for 5 minutes.
5. Garnish with yogurt and chives.

PEA BISQUE WITH FRESH TARRAGON AND SHRIMP

½ pound split peas, rinsed

2-8oz bottles clam juice

6 cups purified water

1 onion, chopped

10 ounces frozen baby peas

1 pound medium shrimp, cleaned

1 tablespoon ghee or butter

6 cloves garlic, crushed

2 tablespoons fresh tarragon leaves, removed from stems

¼ cup white wine

1 tablespoon finely grated lemon zest

1 teaspoon paprika

¼ teaspoon sea salt

1 tablespoon freshly squeezed lemon juice

Tip: One time I had some homemade chipotle sauce left over from a party. I cooked the shrimp in the sauce and then added them to this dish... woo!

1. Place the split peas in a large bowl with enough water to cover. Let stand for 6 hours or overnight.

2. In a large soup pot, place split peas, clam juice, water and onions. Bring to a boil, reduce heat and simmer for 40 minutes.

3. Add thawed peas and simmer for 5 more minutes. Transfer mixture to blender and puree.

4. Saute shrimp and garlic with ghee or butter until shrimp turns pink. Add tarragon, wine, lemon zest, paprika, sea salt and lemon juice. Remove from heat and let stand for 5 minutes.

5. Ladle bisque into shallow soup plates and mound shrimp into center. Garnish with fresh tarragon, a small slice of red pepper and plain yogurt.

Notes from Within: _____

HEALING LEMON GARLIC CHICKEN SOUP

Tip: The garlic, herbs and lemons will cure any cold. Every time I am coming down with something, I drink this soup and all is well.

Notes from Within: _____

2 tablespoons ghee or butter
1 yellow onion, chopped
2 stalks celery, chopped
2 large carrots, peeled and chopped
6 cloves garlic, crushed
8 cups purified water
1 whole free-range chicken
2 tablespoons freshly squeezed lemon juice
1 handful fresh parsley, chopped
1 tablespoon chopped fresh thyme
1 tablespoon chopped fresh oregano
1 tablespoon chopped fresh marjoram
1 tablespoon chopped fresh basil
sea salt and pepper to taste
Optional: 1 cup cooked rice or noodles

1. In a large soup pot, place ghee or butter, onion, celery, carrot and garlic. Brown for 10 minutes.

2. Add water and chicken. Bring to a boil, reduce heat and simmer about 30 minutes. Take chicken out of broth and let cool. Chicken should fall off bone. Separate chicken from bones, then add chicken back into soup.

3. Add lemon juice and fresh herbs, sea salt and pepper to taste, then serve over rice or noodles if desired.

VEGETABLE SOUP

2 tablespoons ghee or butter
4 cloves garlic, crushed
2 yellow onions, chopped
1 cup chopped broccoli
1 cup chopped peeled carrots
1 cup chopped kale
1 cup spinach leaves
1 cup chopped tomato
1 cup string beans
1 cup chopped summer squash
2 tablespoons fresh tarragon leaves, removed from stem
2 teaspoons ground cumin
2 teaspoons chopped fresh rosemary
2 teaspoons chopped fresh sage
8 cups vegetable or chicken stock
2 tablespoons maple syrup
sea salt and cayenne pepper to taste

> *Tip: Sometimes it takes a while before I am satisfied with the taste. I might add soy sauce or red wine to the soup for an extra boost of flavor.*

1. For homemade stock, follow this recipe.

   Vegetable Stock

   3 quarts purified water
   3-4 potatoes, chopped
   3-4 stalks celery, chopped
   4 leaves fresh kale
   6 leaves fresh dandelion
   1 cup dulse (see page 84)

   Bring water to boil in large soup pot. Place vegetables in pot, reduce heat and simmer for 20 minutes. Strain stock. Discard greens and potatoes. Set aside.

2. In a large soup pot, place ghee or butter, garlic and onions. Cook over medium heat until tender.

3. Add broccoli, carrots, kale, spinach, tomato, beans, squash, tarragon, cumin, rosemary, sage and stock. Continue to cook for 20 minutes.

4. Add maple syrup, sea salt and cayenne pepper to season.

Notes from Within: _____

POTLATCH STEW

Tip: I have read this stew is made for Tribal Celebrations and served on special occasions such as marriage, the naming of a child or building a house.

Notes from Within: _____

2 tablespoons unrefined coconut oil
1 onion, diced
1 bulb fennel, diced
3 large carrots, peeled and chopped
2 tablespoons chopped fresh cilantro
2 tablespoons chopped fresh thyme
2 tablespoons chopped fresh basil
2 tablespoons chopped fresh mint
2 tablespoons tomato paste
4 fresh tomatoes, chopped
1 cup purified water
½ teaspoon sea salt
8 ounces halibut
8 ounces salmon, skinned
10 prawns, de-veined
10 sea scallops
1 ½ cups white wine
12 green mussels in shell, cleaned
12 manila clams in shell, cleaned
4 crab legs

1. Heat coconut oil in a large soup pot. Add onion, fennel, carrots, cilantro, thyme, basil and mint. Saute vegetables for 5 minutes over medium heat. Add tomato paste and cook for another 4 minutes.

2. Add tomatoes, water and sea salt to pot. Bring to a boil, reduce heat and simmer for 25 minutes.

3. Add halibut, salmon, prawns and scallops to stew. Simmer over medium heat for 5 minutes or until seafood is cooked.

4. In a separate saucepan, bring wine to a boil. Add clams and mussels. Cover and cook until opened. Remember to shake pan to help open shells. Add crab legs and finish cooking for 5 minutes. Add to soup and serve!

BLACK BEAN SOUP

3 tablespoons unrefined coconut oil
1 yellow onion, chopped
6 cloves garlic, crushed
1 large celery stalk, chopped
1 large carrot, chopped
2 teaspoons ground cumin
4 cups free-range chicken or vegetable stock
3-15½ oz. cans all natural organic black beans, rinsed and drained.
1 tablespoon tomato paste
2 teaspoons freshly squeezed lime juice
maple syrup and sea salt to taste

> Tip: Garnish with plain yogurt, salsa, cilantro and blue corn chips. Once I placed large pawns in the soup bowl with the tails sticking up out of the soup. Great presentation and it tasted good too!

1. In a large pot, sauté onion and garlic in coconut oil. Cook until tender. Add celery and carrots. Stir in cumin, cook for 10 minutes.

2. Add stock and beans to the pot. Bring soup to a boil, then reduce heat, cover and simmer for 20 minutes.

3. Add tomato paste and lime juice to soup. Puree in blender and add sea salt to taste. A tablespoon of maple syrup will make the soup come alive!

Notes from Within: _____
_____
_____
_____
_____
_____
_____
_____
_____
_____
_____
_____
_____

CELERY ROOT SOUP

Notes from Within: _____

4 tablespoons ghee or butter

1 yellow onion, diced

5 cloves garlic, crushed

2 large celery roots, peeled and cut into ½ inch cubes

2 quarts chicken stock

1 bunch fresh parsley, chopped

sea salt and cayenne pepper to taste

6 tablespoons dry sherry

1. In a large soup pot, sauté onion, garlic and celery roots in ghee or butter until tender.
2. Add stock, bring to a boil, reduce heat and simmer for 40 minutes.
3. Puree mixture and return to pot.
4. Add parsley and seasonings. One tablespoon of sherry can be added to individual bowls. Garnish with a swirl of cream.

CUCUMBER KEFIR/YOGURT SOUP

1 large cucumber, peeled and diced
1 cup plain kefir
1 tablespoon freshly squeezed lemon juice
½ cup chopped fresh dill
2 cloves garlic, crushed
1 teaspoon soy sauce

1. In a blender, combine cucumber, kefir, lemon, dill and garlic.
2. Season with soy sauce.
3. Chill in refrigerator, then serve.

> *Tip: This is a great cool soup for hot summer days. I hope you like garlic! It's "very garlicy."*

Notes from Within: _____

_____
_____
_____
_____
_____
_____
_____
_____
_____
_____
_____
_____

SWEET POTATO AND ROSEMARY SOUP

Notes from Within: _____

1 tablespoon unrefined coconut oil
1 large white onion, chopped
3 large cloves garlic, crushed
6 cups free-range chicken broth
4 cups cubed sweet potatoes
1 cup soy milk
1 tablespoon chopped fresh rosemary
1 tablespoon cayenne pepper
1 teaspoon sea salt

1. In a large pot, sauté onions and garlic in oil until light brown.
2. Add broth and sweet potatoes to pot and bring to boil. Reduce heat and cover. Simmer for 30 minutes.
3. Puree cooked mixture and return to pot on low heat.
4. Add milk, rosemary, cayenne pepper and sea salt. Garnish with a sprig of rosemary.

RED CURRY LENTIL SOUP

❄

2 tablespoons ghee or butter
1 large onion, chopped
3 large cloves garlic, crushed
4 tablespoons curry powder
1 tablespoon cumin seeds
½ cup chopped peeled carrots
½ cup chopped potatoes
6 cups chicken stock
1 ½ cups red lentils, cleaned and rinsed
2 tablespoons maple syrup
1 tablespoon soy sauce
½ cup chopped fresh cilantro

1. In a large soup pot, sauté onion and garlic in ghee or butter until tender.

2. Add curry powder, cumin seeds, carrots and potatoes, cook for 10 more minutes.

3. Add stock, lentils, maple syrup, soy sauce and cilantro. Bring to a boil, reduce heat and simmer for 20 minutes.

Notes from Within: _____

WILD MUSHROOM SOUP

☼ ❄

Tip: I serve the soup in a shallow soup bowl and place watermelon carrots (or garlic mashed potatoes) in the middle of the soup. I top the dish with strips of mustard chicken with fresh thyme. This is an unusual dish, but got great reviews when served.

Notes from Within: _____

_____
_____
_____
_____
_____
_____
_____
_____
_____
_____

2 tablespoons ghee or butter

8 cloves garlic, crushed

3 leeks, (white and light green parts only), cleaned and chopped

2 pounds mushrooms (button, crimini, shiitake, porcini, Portabella and chanterelle), brushed clean

1 cup sherry

4 tablespoons soy sauce

6 cups chicken stock

2 tablespoons heavy cream

¼ cup chopped fresh parsley

1. In a soup pot, sauté garlic, leeks and mushrooms in ghee or butter until tender. Add sherry and soy sauce. Cook 1 more minute over medium heat.

2. Add stock, bring to a boil, reduce heat and simmer for 20 minutes.

3. Before serving, add cream and parsley.

2 cups chopped roasted chestnuts
7 cups chicken stock
¼ cup apple cider
6 shallots
1 tablespoon olive oil
2 tablespoons honey
½ teaspoon chopped fresh sage
½ cup dry white wine
¼ cup soy milk
sea salt and pepper to taste

1. Cook chestnuts, stock and cider in a large pot over medium heat for 30 minutes or until chestnuts are soft.

2. While you are waiting, brush each shallot with olive oil and bake at 375°F for 50 minutes. Remove from oven and cool.

3. Transfer chestnut mixture to food processor or blender. Add honey, shallots and sage. Process until mixture is creamy.

4. Transfer soup back into pot and add milk. Season with sea salt and pepper to taste.

5. Garnish with yogurt and a fresh sprig of sage. Top with pomegranate seeds.

CHESTNUTS ROASTING ON AN OPEN FIRE SOUP

Tip: The roasting ceremony could be really fun if you had a group of people around the fire. I found myself roasting chestnuts in the oven set at 400°F. Cut into each chestnut with a knife making an X. Bake for 10-20 minutes and as the chestnuts bake, the X begins to open. Make sure you use gloves. (This adventure could be hard on your fingerprints.) Peel the shells and let cool.

Notes from Within: _____

5 MINUTE SOUP

> Tip: Add a little lemon. This is a great cleansing soup.

Notes from Within: _____

1 tablespoon olive oil
2 cloves garlic, crushed
6 cups chicken stock
½ cup fresh peas
½ cup chopped peeled carrots
½ cup asparagus tips
1 cup fresh spinach leaves
½ teaspoon cayenne pepper
½ teaspoon sea salt

1. In a soup pot, sauté garlic in oil until brown.
2. Add chicken stock, peas, carrots, asparagus and spinach to pot.
3. Cook soup 5 minutes so vegetables are still crunchy. Season with cayenne pepper and sea salt.
4. If you have extra time cook rice and add to soup.

SMOKED SALMON AND CREAM CHEESE SOUP

½ cup ghee or butter
2 medium yellow onions, chopped
1 cup chopped fresh dill weed
8-10 ounces smoked salmon, finely chopped
2 medium tomatoes, chopped
2 tablespoons spelt flour
8 cups purified water
2 cups fresh spinach leaves
2-8oz packages cream cheese
⅓ cup vodka
4 tablespoons freshly squeezed lemon juice
freshly ground black pepper to taste
chives to garnish

1. In a stock pot, sauté onions in butter until tender.
2. Stir in dill, salmon and tomatoes. Cook for 5 minutes more and add flour.
3. Gradually stir in water. Heat until boiling, reduce heat and simmer uncovered for 20 minutes.
4. Stir in spinach and cream cheese. Over low heat, stir to a creamy texture.
5. Add vodka and lemon juice. Season to taste. Garnish with chives.

Tip: A student came to class offering me a large slab of smoked salmon. She had a family gathering and it was leftover. Here is a very rich and hearty soup perfect for a cold winter day.

Notes from Within: _____

CARROT GINGER SOUP

> Tip: I use 3 bags of already cleaned baby carrots. It just makes the cooking process go faster!

Notes from Within: _____

½ cup ghee or butter

1 large yellow onion, chopped

¼ cup chopped fresh ginger root

6 cloves garlic, crushed

7 cups free-range chicken stock

1 cup dry white wine

1 ½ pounds carrots, peeled and chopped into ½ inch pieces

2 tablespoons freshly squeezed lemon juice

2 tablespoons curry powder

sea salt to taste

cayenne pepper to taste

A dash of stevia (herb) or 1 tablespoon maple syrup

1. Melt butter in a large stock pot over medium heat. Add onion, ginger and garlic. Saute for 20 minutes.

2. Add stock, wine and carrots. Bring to a boil and reduce heat. Simmer until carrots are tender, about 45 minutes.

3. Add lemon juice and curry powder, then puree the soup in a blender. Season to taste with sea salt, cayenne pepper and stevia or maple syrup.

Breakfast

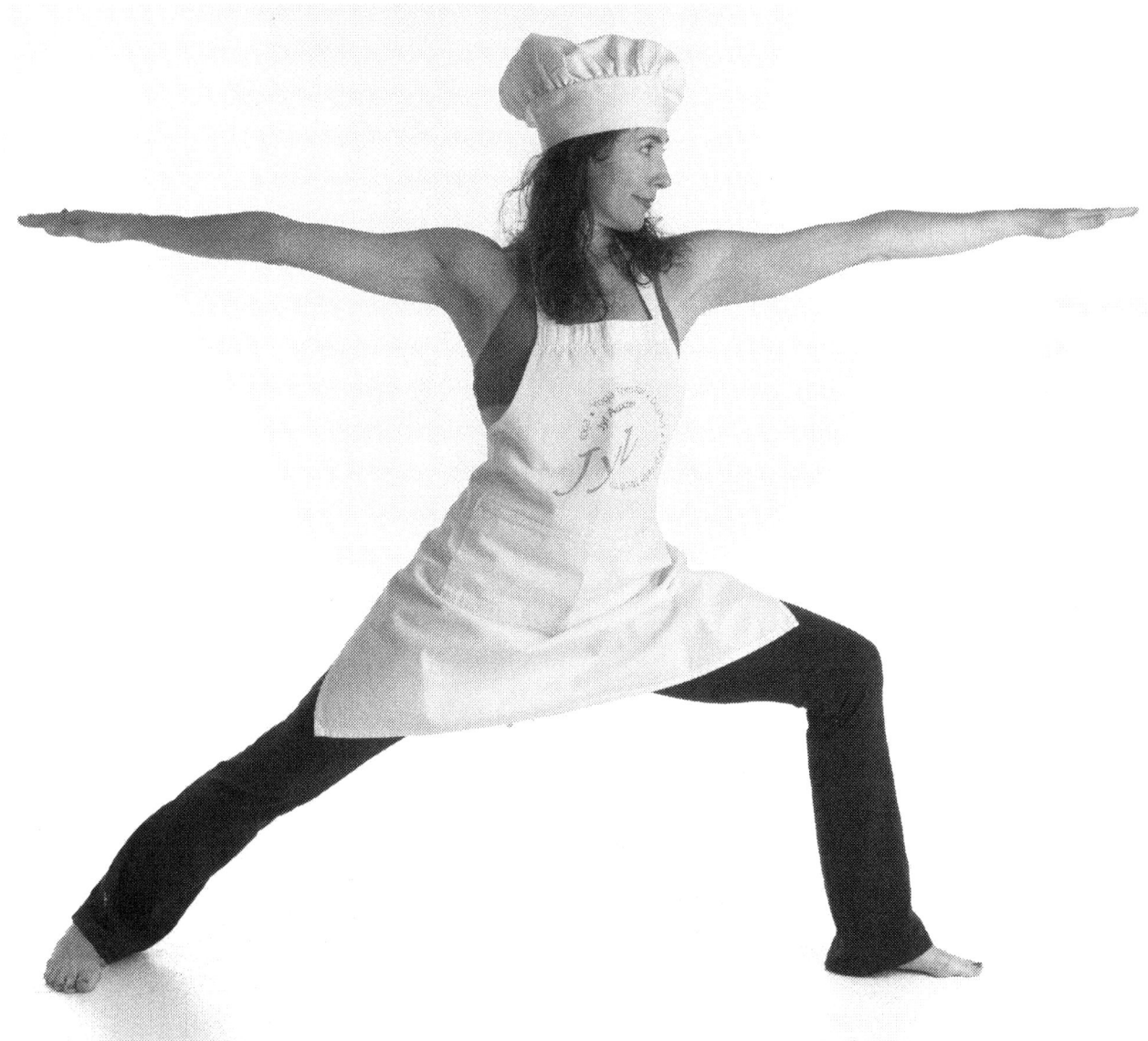

PANCAKES

¼ cup melted butter or ghee
2 cups oat flour
½ teaspoon sea salt
2 teaspoons baking powder (aluminum-free)
2 free-range eggs
1 cup purified water

Notes from Within: _____

1. Melt butter in pan.
2. Combine flour, sea salt and baking powder in a glass bowl and add melted butter.
3. Whisk in eggs and water.
4. For lighter pancakes separate egg whites and beat separately, then fold into mixture.
5. Pour batter into hot oiled pan. Cook until golden brown on each side.
6. Top cakes with fresh fruit, yogurt, and maple syrup.

FRENCH TOAST

5 eggs

¼ cup heavy cream

2 tablespoons vanilla

2 teaspoons ground cinnamon

2 teaspoons ground cloves

4-6 slices bread (wheat-free and yeast-free)

2 tablespoons ghee or butter

⅓ cup walnuts

Optional: strawberry jam, maple syrup, and yogurt

> *Tip: I use rice bread that you can buy at a local health food store. This sweet bread makes wonerful french toast! Plus it is gluten free, perfect for my healthy body.*

1. Combine eggs, cream, vanilla, cinnamon and cloves and whisk.
2. Cover each slice of bread with egg mixture.
3. In saucepan, heat ghee or butter and walnuts. Brown the nuts until golden.
4. Place slices of bread directly on top of nuts and brown French toast. Serve this nutty breakfast treat with a spoonful of strawberry jam and yogurt. Top with warm maple syrup.

Notes from Within: _____

LOVE YOURSELF SCRAMBLED EGGS

Tip: Usually, my breakfast is a piece of fruit or kefir. In the wintertime my Vatta is off balance and I need warm foods. These eggs really feed my soul.

Notes from Within: _____

_____
_____
_____
_____
_____
_____
_____
_____
_____
_____
_____
_____

Scramble for one:

1 teaspoon ghee or butter
2 cloves garlic, crushed
3 stalks asparagus, chopped
1 medium carrot, peeled and chopped
1 cup fresh peas
1 cup fresh baby arugula leaves
2 free-range eggs
½ cup daikon radish sprouts
¼ cup sunflower sprouts
1 teaspoon flax seed oil
1 tablespoon chopped fresh mint

1. In a medium size saucepan, melt ghee or butter.

2. Saute garlic, followed by asparagus, carrot, peas and arugula. Cook for 5 minutes. Add eggs to vegetables and scramble.

3. Drizzle flaxseed oil slowly over entire dish and top with sprouts and mint. Garnish with a sprig of fresh mint and you have a wonderful meal.

KEFIR

For hot summer months try a new breakfast idea. Kefir is a cultured, microbial-rich food whose strains of bacteria make it a powerful natural antibiotic. This type of food is great for the colon. Kefir is like yogurt, however the difference between them is the way they are made. Yogurt is made with heat, so it is considered not as beneficial as kefir, which is made naturally without the heating process. If you want to make your own, just add a starter culture of bacteria (acidophilus or bifidus powder) to room-temperature raw milk. Let stand out on the counter in your kitchen for 24 hours, then refrigerate. If you are using goat's milk, you will need more culture. Instead of one package use one and a half packets.

> *Tip: I also will add my super greens to the kefir. It tastes great, just looks a little weird and very green.*

1 cup plain or vanilla kefir (most health food stores will carry)

1 handful blue berries, green apples, nuts (soaked almonds page 70), raw pumpkin seeds and sunflower seeds

1 tablespoon maple, strawberry or coffee flavorings

1 tablespoon crushed flaxseeds

stevia (herbal sweetener) to taste

garnish with a fresh sprig of mint

Notes from Within: _____

Breads

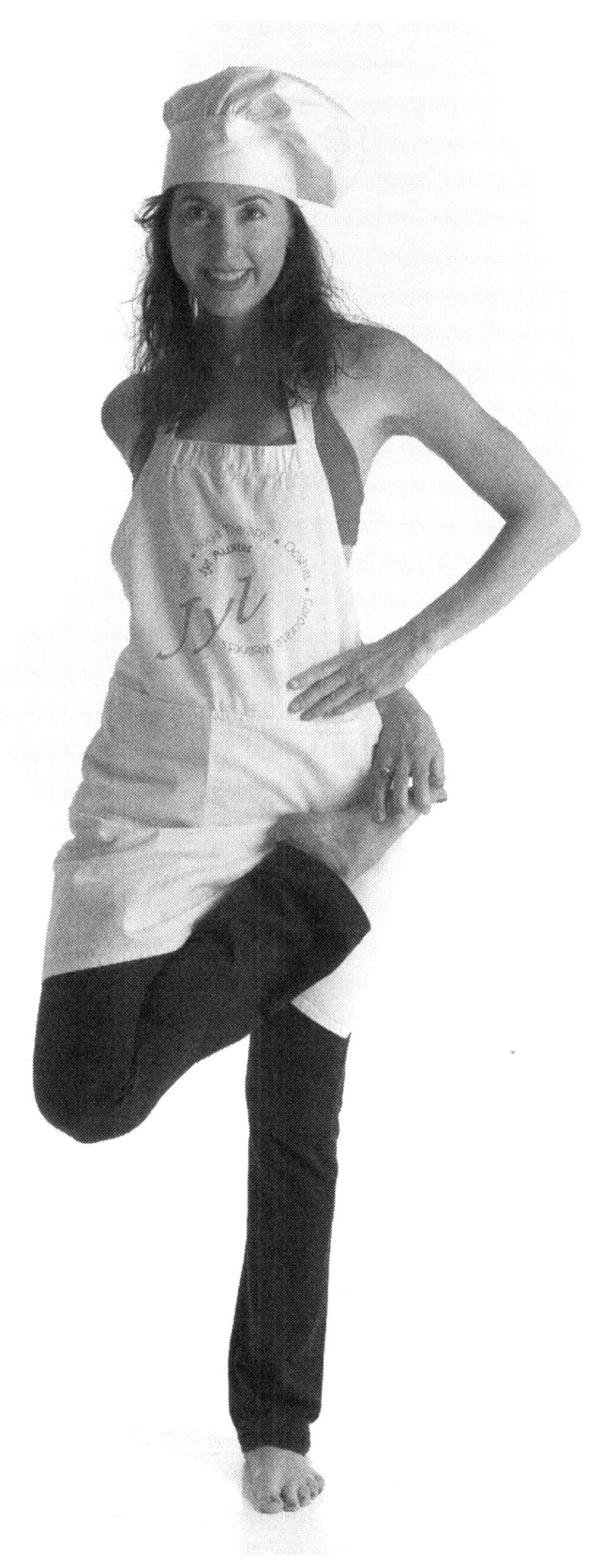

GOAT-CHEESE POPOVERS

Tip: If you use white flour, the muffins will look bigger and more like a popover. The soy flour is denser and the muffins look more like little hockey pucks, but taste wonderful.

Notes from Within: _____

6 free-range eggs
1 ½ cups soy flour
dash sea salt
dash freshly grounded pepper
1 cup soy milk
½ cup whipping cream
1 tablespoon chopped fresh thyme
1 tablespoon fresh tarragon leaves, removed from stem
1 tablespoon chopped fresh rosemary
1 tablespoon chopped fresh parsley
4 ounces herbed chavrie, cut into 12 pieces

1. Preheat oven to 400°F.

2. Brush tins for 12 muffins with oil. Place muffin tins in oven and heat for 5 minutes.

3. In a blender, place eggs, flour, sea salt, pepper, soy milk, whipping cream, thyme, tarragon, rosemary and parsley and blend until fully mixed.

4. Take empty hot tins from oven and fill each muffin cup ⅔ full with mixture. Place herbed chavrie into each muffin cup.

5. Place tins back into hot oven and bake for 20-30 minutes.

BLUEBERRY CORN MUFFINS

1 cup cornmeal
1 cup oat flour
⅓ cup maple syrup
2 ½ teaspoons baking powder
dash sea salt
1 cup soy milk
6 tablespoons melted ghee or butter
1 free-range egg
2 cups fresh or frozen blueberries

1. Preheat oven to 400°F and rub tins for 12 muffins with oil.
2. Combine cornmeal, flour, maple syrup, baking powder and sea salt. Mix.
3. Stir in milk, ghee or butter and egg.
4. Fold in berries.
5. Fill each muffin cup ⅔ full. Bake for 20 minutes.

Notes from Within: _____

PUMPKIN-ALMOND BREAD

> Tip: I call this my Goddess Bread. This is one of the most delicious breads I have ever encountered. Enjoy!
>
> Very Important: Test this bread to see if it is done by placing a wooden skewer in the middle. If it comes up clean, the bread is baked.

Notes from Within: _____

¼ cup melted ghee or butter
1 cup spelt flour
¾ cup almond butter
½ teaspoon baking powder
1 teaspoon baking soda
½ teaspoon sea salt
2 teaspoons ground cinnamon
2 teaspoons ground cloves
2 teaspoons ground nutmeg
2 teaspoons ground ginger
¾ cup maple syrup
2 free-range eggs
1-15oz jar organic pumpkin pie filling
⅓ cup soy milk
¼ cup dried black currents
¼ cup pumpkin seeds

1. Preheat oven to 350°F and grease a 9" glass bread pan.

2. In a large bowl, combine butter or ghee, flour and almond butter. Mix together. Add baking powder, baking soda, sea salt, cinnamon, cloves, nutmeg, ginger, maple syrup, eggs, pumpking pie filling, soy milk, black currants and pumpkin seeds. Mix well.

3. Pour into bread pan and bake for 40-50 minutes. This bread is very moist. Make sure bread is done before removing from oven.

Desserts

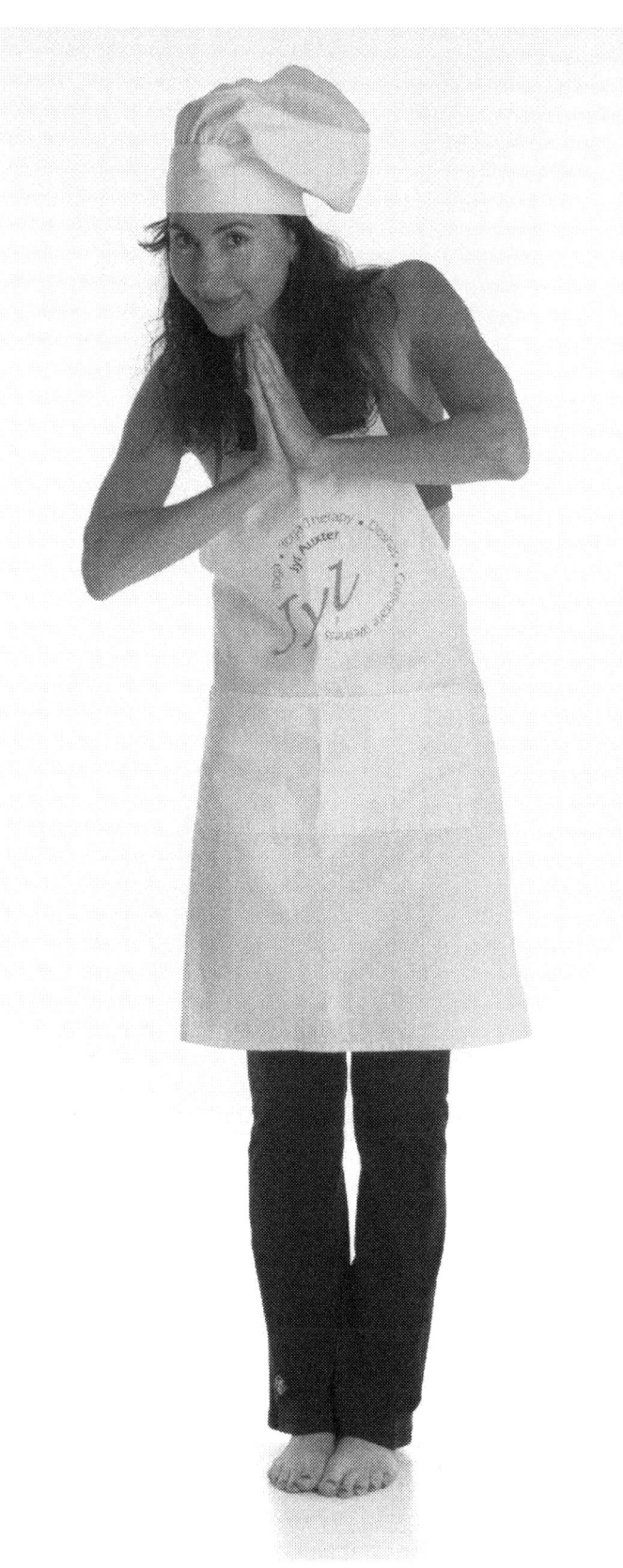

LEMON-LIME TOFU CREME PIE

Tip: Interesting new dessert. Serve with strawberry sauce and a sprig of mint.

Notes from Within: _____

Crust:

- 4 tablespoons melted ghee or butter
- 1 ½ tablespoons honey
- ¾ cup raw oats
- 2 tablespoons sesame seeds
- ¼ cup oat flour
- ¼ teaspoon sea salt
- ¼ teaspoon cinnamon
- 2 tablespoons minced walnuts or almonds
- ¼ teaspoon vanilla

Filling:

- 23 ounces firm tofu, chopped
- ⅓ cup freshly squeezed lemon juice
- ¼ cup freshly squeezed lime juice
- ⅔ cup honey
- ⅓ cup olive oil
- 2 teaspoons vanilla
- 2 teaspoons ground ginger
- ⅛ teaspoon sea salt
- 1 tablespoon cornstarch

1. *To prepare crust:* In a large bowl, combine ghee or butter and honey, then add oats, sesame seeds, flour, sea salt, cinnamon walnuts or almonds and vanilla. Mix well.

2. Press the crust into a 9-inch round pie pan.

3. Preheat the oven to 350°F.

4. *To prepare filling:* In a blender, combine tofu, lemon juice, lime juice, honey, olive oil, vanilla, ginger, sea salt and cornstarch. Blend until very smooth.

5. Place filling into crust and bake for 30 minutes.

6. Chill and serve with sliced almonds or walnuts.

CAROB ALMOND COOKIES

1 ½ large apples or pears, chopped
⅓ cup almond butter
¼ cup ghee or butter, melted
2 free-range eggs
¼ teaspoon vitamin C crystals
1 ¼ cups oat flour
¼ cup spelt flour
¾ teaspoon baking soda
¾ cup carob powder
¼ teaspoon sea salt
20 whole almonds, soaked (page 70)

1. Preheat oven 350°F.

2. In blender, place chopped apples or pears, almond butter, ghee or butter, eggs and vitamin C crystals. Puree. Add water to mixture if needed.

3. Combine flour, baking soda, carob powder and sea salt in a bowl and add puree. Stir well.

4. Drop tablespoon size cookie dough on greased cookie sheet. Top each cookie with an almond. Bake 10-12 minutes.

> *Tip: This is a great cookie for someone with a restrictive diet. Children love these cookies, believe it or not. You can add 2 tablespoons of maple syrup to the recipe to sweeten.*
>
> *Yeast and sugar free!*

Notes from Within: _____

GREEN TEA POACHED PEARS

4 cups purified water

6-8 Jasmine Green Tea bags or 4 tablespoons loose tea

1 cup freshly squeezed orange juice

1 tablespoon maple syrup

½ teaspoon vanilla

1 tablespoon port wine

2 tablespoons strawberry jam

2 Bartlett pears, peeled, halved and cored

> Tip: Serve hot with your favorite ice cream. Throw some pistachios nuts on top and make sure you include the left over sauce with each serving.

1. Heat water and let tea steep for 5 minutes.

2. In a saucepan, combine tea, orange juice, maple syrup, vanilla, port wine and jam.

3. Bring mixture to a boil and gently add pear halves. Make sure mixture covers pears. Simmer for 20 minutes and serve.

Notes from Within: _____

BALSAMIC ROASTED PEARS WITH GOAT CHEESE

¼ cup unsalted ghee or butter
3 firm-ripe Bosc pears, halved and cored
4 tablespoons balsamic vinegar
6 slices goat cheese
½ cup honey

1. Preheat oven to 400 °F.
2. Place butter in an 8-inch square baking dish and melt in oven for 5 minutes.
3. Slice pears in half, place cut side down in melted butter and bake for 20 minutes.
4. Pour balsamic vinegar over pears and roast for 5 more minutes.
5. Serve pears on plate with cheese. Drizzle pears and cheese with honey

Notes from Within: _____

FOR CHOCOLATE LOVERS CHOCOLATE CREPES WITH STRAWBERRY FILLING

Tip: This is a light summer dessert that can be made up well in advance. The strawberries must be organic!!!

Notes from Within: _____

Crepe:

1 cup oat flour

2 tablespoons cocoa powder

1 free-range egg yolk

1 ¾ cups soy milk

1 tablespoon olive oil

Filling:

3 cups thinly sliced fresh strawberries

2 tablespoons maple syrup

2 tablespoons freshly squeezed lemon juice

1. *To prepare crepe batter:* Combine oat flour, cocoa, egg yolk, milk and olive oil. Mix well and chill for 30 minutes.

2. *To prepare filling:* Clean and slice strawberries and place in saucepan. Add syrup and lemon juice, cook on low heat for 20 minutes.

3. On a heated nonstick grill, or if you have a crepe pan, pour batter thinly. Cook crepes on each side until golden brown.

4. Fill crepe with strawberry filling and top with whipping cream and your favorite liqueur.

STRAWBERRY OATMEAL CAKE

Oatmeal Cake:

- ½ cup room temperature ghee or butter
- 1 cup sucanat sugar
- ½ cup maple syrup
- ½ cup brown sugar
- 2 cups boiling water
- 1 ½ cups rolled oats
- 2 free-range eggs
- 1 teaspoon vanilla
- 1 ⅓ cups oat flour
- 1 teaspoon baking soda
- 1 teaspoon sea salt
- 2 teaspoons ground cinnamon
- 2 teaspoons ground nutmeg

Strawberry Topping:

- *2 cups freshly cut strawberries (organic is a must)*
- *¼ cup watermelon juice*
- *½ cup maple syrup*
- *½ cup dark rum*
- *1 tablespoon lemon juice*

> Tip: Use this recipe to replace your strawberry shortcake. It gets better with age... Don't we all... if you cook like I do, a dessert that you can make a day or two before your event comes in handy.

1. *To prepare cake:* Preheat oven to 350°F. Grease 9x13 inch pan

2. In a large mixing bowl, cream ghee or butter, sugar, maple syrup and brown sugar. Blend with a mixer on medium speed until smooth.

3. In a separate bowl, add boiling water to oats and set aside.

4. Add eggs, vanilla, flour, baking soda, sea salt, cinnamon and nutmeg to sugar and butter mixture. Add oats to mixing bowl and mix well. Pour batter into baking pan and bake for 20 minutes.

5. *To prepare topping:* Clean and slice strawberries.

6. In a saucepan, combine strawberries, watermelon juice, maple syrup, rum and lemon juice. Bring to a boil. Reduce heat and simmer for 20 minutes.

Notes from Within: _____

BEET CAKE WITH CREAM CHEESE FROSTING

Notes from Within: _____

Cake:

1 pound beets

⅔ cup sucanat sugar

⅔ cup maple syrup

½ cup olive oil

2 free-range eggs

½ cup soy milk

2 ½ cups oat flour

2 teaspoons baking powder

1 teaspoon ground ginger

1 teaspoon ground cinnamon

½ teaspoon baking soda

¼ teaspoon sea salt

Frosting:

2 teaspoons grated orange rind

1 teaspoon vanilla extract

1-8oz package cream cheese

3 cups sifted powdered sugar

2 tablespoons chopped walnuts

1. *To prepare cake:* Preheat oven to 350°F and grease one 9 inch round cake pan.

2. Peel and grate beets. Measure 2 cups of beets.

3. Combine sugar, syrup, oil, eggs and milk. Mix well.

4. Add beets and stir well before adding flour, baking powder, ginger, cinnamon, baking soda and sea salt.

5. Pour batter in pan and bake for 30 minutes.

6. *To prepare frosting:* While cake is baking, beat orange rind, vanilla and cream cheese together with a mixer at high speed, until fluffy.

7. Add powdered sugar, beat on low just until blended (do not over beat). Mix in walnuts. When the cake is cooled, frost!

GINGERBREAD CAKE

2 cups oat flour
2 teaspoons ground ginger
2 teaspoons ground cinnamon
1 teaspoon baking powder
1 teaspoon baking soda
½ teaspoon sea salt
½ teaspoon ground cloves
¾ cup buttermilk
¼ cup soy milk
½ cup maple syrup
1 cup molasses
¼ cup room temperature butter
2 large free-range eggs
1 cup fresh blueberries

1. Preheat oven to 350°F and grease 9-inch square baking pan.
2. In a large bowl, mix together flour, ginger, cinnamon, baking powder, baking soda, sea salt, cloves, buttermilk, soy milk, maple syrup, molassas, butter, eggs and blueberries.
3. Pour batter into baking pan and bake for 45 minutes.
4. Top the cake with your favorite icing or fresh fruit and frozen yogurt.

Notes from Within: _____

CHOCOLATE PUDDING CAKE

> Tip: This dish must be served hot with ice cream and drizzled with chocolate. "Very Naughty!"

Notes from Within: _____

⅓ cup unsweetened chocolate
½ cup melted unsalted butter
1 ⅓ cups sucanat sugar
1 cup soy flour
1 ½ teaspoons baking powder
½ teaspoon sea salt
½ cup soy milk
½ cup dark brown sugar
3 tablespoons unsweetened cocoa
2 teaspoons vanilla
2 tablespoons rum
1 ½ cups boiling water

1. Preheat oven to 350°F. Grease a 9-inch square pan.
2. In a double boiler, melt chocolate.
3. Combine butter and half of sucanat sugar. Add flour, baking powder, sea salt and mix in milk.
4. Fold melted chocolate into mixture and pour into pan.
5. In a separate bowl, stir remaining sugar, brown sugar and cocoa. Sprinkle over batter in pan.
6. Bring water to a boil and add vanilla and rum. Pour water slowly over batter. Bake for an hour.

WHITE CHOCOLATE CHEESECAKE

Tip: I usually garnish the plate with a freshly cooked strawberry sauce. Place this light and fluffy cheesecake in a pool of strawberry sauce, and top with one large organic strawberry and a sprig of mint. 10 servings.

Crust:

    4 tablespoons melted ghee or butter

    1 ½ tablespoons honey

    ¾ cup raw oats

    2 tablespoons sesame seeds

    ¼ cup oat flour

    ¼ teaspoon sea salt

    ¼ teaspoon ground cinnamon

    2 tablespoons minced walnuts or almonds

    ¼ teaspoon vanilla

Filling:

    10 ounces white chocolate

    ½ cup heavy cream

    1 pound cream cheese

    ½ cup sucanat sugar

    4 large free-range egg yolks

    1 tablespoon vanilla

    4 large free-range egg whites

1. *To prepare crust:* In a large bowl, Combine ghee or butter and honey. Then add oats, sesame seeds, flour, sea salt, cinnamon, nuts and vanilla.

2. Press the crust into a greased spring form pan.

3. *To prepare filling:* Place chocolate and cream in a double boiler and melt.

4. In a separate mixing bowl, combine cream cheese, sugar and egg yolks. Beat with mixer on medium to high setting until smooth.

5. When chocolate has melted and cooled, add to cream cheese mixture, then add vanilla.

6. In a separate bowl, whip egg whites on high speed until stiff. Fold ½ of egg whites into mixture and stir gently until well mixed. Fold in remaining whites. Be sure not to deflate.

7. Bake for 50 minutes at 325°F. Turn off oven but let cake stand in oven with the door closed for 1 hour.

Notes from Within: _____

CHOCOLATE TRUFFLE TART

> Tip: Very rich dessert so plan on serving small slices. Drizzle with chocolate or raspberry sauce.

Notes from Within: _____

Crust:

1 ½ cups hazelnuts, finely ground
¼ cup sucanat sugar
½ cup melted butter

Filling:

12 ounces semisweet chocolate
8 tablespoons butter
4 free-range egg yolks
¼ cup sucanat sugar
½ cup heavy cream or cream substitute
2 tablespoons dark rum

1. *To prepare crust:* Preheat oven to 450°F and grease spring form pan.

2. In a mixing bowl, combine hazelnuts, sugar and butter. Mix well.

3. In a greased spring form pan, press mixture to make crust. Bake for 5 minutes.

4. *To prepare filling:* Using a double boiler, melt 8 ounces of chopped chocolate and butter. Stir until smooth and set aside to cool.

5. Place egg yolks and sugar in a mixing bowl and beat with electric mixer until thick ribbons form.

6. Add egg mixture to chocolate and whisk over low heat for 3-4 minutes. The mixture should reach 145°F. Pour mixture into crust.

7. In a saucepan, heat cream on medium heat and add remaining chocolate. Stir until melted and smooth. Stir in rum and pour mixture over tart.

8. Refrigerate for 2 hours. Garnish with raspberries.

CHOCOLATE GANACHE SAUCE

1 cup heavy cream or soy milk

1 package semisweet chocolate chips or tofu chocolate chips

1. Combine liquid and chips in a double boiler and melt.
2. Stir mixture until fully melted and smooth.
3. Drizzle chocolate in middle of cake and let drip down the cake.

> *Tip. I use this instead of frosting for all my desserts. This sauce is easy and delicious.*
>
> *For anyone who loves chocolate with peppermint, try adding natural alcohol free peppermint flavoring to your ganache sauce.*

Notes from Within: _____

_____
_____
_____
_____
_____
_____
_____
_____

CHOCOLATE TORT

8 ounces bittersweet chocolate

¾ cup room temperature butter or ghee

¾ cup sucanat sugar

6 extra-large free-range eggs yolks

1 ½ cups ground walnuts or hazelnuts

6 extra-large free-range eggs whites

> Tip: This is a very rich and impressive dessert. Perfect for afternoon tea. Serves 10.

1. Preheat oven 350°F. Grease a 10-inch layer cake pan or spring form pan with 3-inch sides. Line bottom of pan with parchment paper or waxed paper.

2. Place chocolate in a double boiler and melt. Stir until the chocolate is melted and smooth. Set aside to cool.

3. In another bowl, combine butter and sugar. Beat until light and fluffy with a mixer. Add egg yolks one at a time. Beat in the cooled chocolate and ground nuts.

4. Beat egg whites until stiff and glossy. Using a spatula, gently fold egg whites into mixture.

5. Pour mixture into pan and bake for 50 minutes.

6. Cool tort and top with chocolate ganache sauce (page 176).

Notes from Within: _____

JYL'S FAMOUS TOFU BIRTHDAY CAKE

2 ¼ cups oat flour
2 teaspoons baking powder
½ teaspoon sea salt
1 ¼ cups sucanat sugar
½ cup room temperature butter
8 ounces soft tofu
1 ½ cups soy milk
2 teaspoons vanilla
½ cup strawberry jam
1 pint fresh strawberries, thinly sliced

1. Preheat oven to 350°F. Grease two 8-inch cake pans.
2. In a large bowl, combine flour, baking powder and sea salt. Set aside.
3. In another mixing bowl, mix sugar and butter until creamy.
4. In a food processor or blender, mix tofu, soy milk and vanilla until smooth. Combine tofu and sugar mixtures. Add liquid mixture to dry ingredients.
5. Pour batter into pans and bake for 30 minutes.
6. Cool cakes to room temperature. Place one cake layer on serving plate and evenly spread strawberry jam and freshly sliced strawberries on top. Place second cake layer over first and frost with chocolate ganache sauce (page 176).

Tip: People love this cake!!! You can expect to get 10 servings.

Notes from Within: _____

POMEGRANATE SOY ICE CREAM

1 cup watermelon juice
½ cup unrefined cane sugar
1 ½ cups pomegranate juice
2 cups soy milk or whole milk
½ cup pomegranate seeds

Notes from Within: _____

1. In a saucepan, heat watermelon juice over medium heat for 10 minutes.
2. Add sugar and pomegranate juice. Cook 10 minutes more.
3. Refrigerate until chilled.
4. Combine chilled juice mixture and milk. Process in an ice cream maker until thick, or about 15 minutes.
5. Add pomegranate seeds and finish processing.

Sauces & Salad Dressings

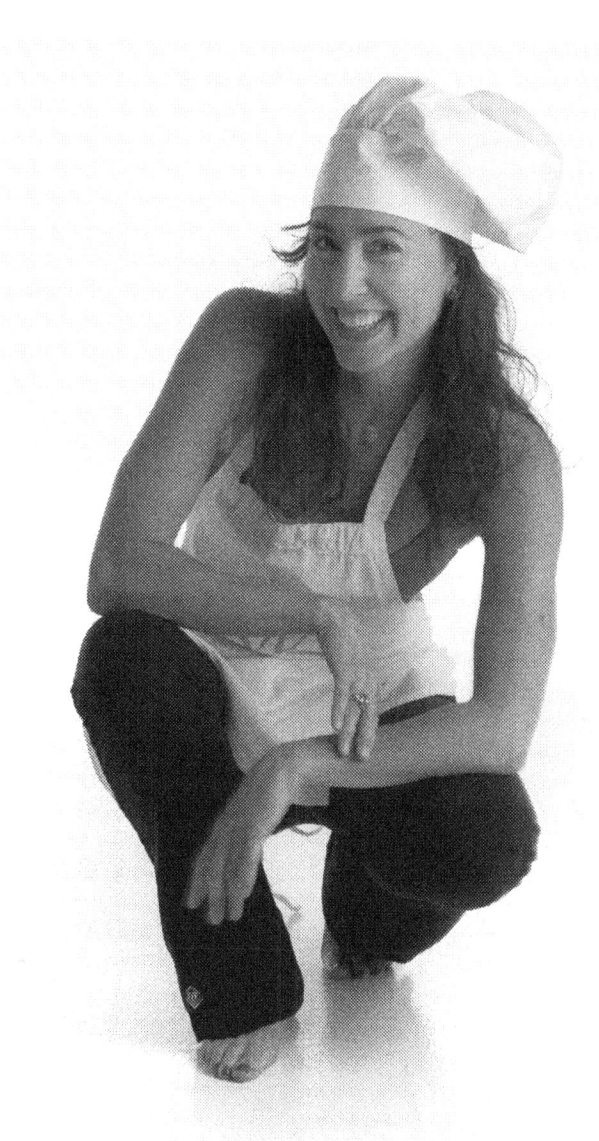

MINT-GARLIC SALAD DRESSING

Notes from Within: _____

1/4 cup fresh lemon juice
1 tablespoon minced fresh mint leaves
3 cloves garlic, minced
1/2 cup olive oil

1. Combine lemon juice, mint and garlic in a blender.
2. Blend, slowly add oil to emulsify.

MUSTARD BASIL SALAD DRESSING

½ cup chopped fresh basil
3 cloves garlic, crushed
2 tablespoons Dijon-style mustard
¼ cup balsamic vinegar
2 cups olive oil
2 tablespoons lemon juice
1 tablespoon maple syrup
1 teaspoon cayenne pepper

1. Combine and chop fresh basil and garlic.
2. In a blender, combine basil, garlic, mustard, vinegar and oil. Blend.
3. Add lemon juice, maple syrup and cayenne pepper.

Notes from Within: _____

BASIL PESTO

Tip: The amount of olive oil will depend how you like your pesto. I usually like mine a little oilier.

Notes from Within: _____

¾ cup chopped fresh basil
1 teaspoon sea salt
¼ cup Parmesan cheese
3 cloves garlic, crushed
½ cup whole pine nuts
¼ cup olive oil

1. Clean and chop fresh basil. Combine with sea salt, Parmesan cheese, garlic, pine nuts and oil in food processor.
2. Blend until texture is smooth.

SAUCY SAUCES FOR SASSY STUDENTS

✿ ☼ ❄

Most of my dishes include some sauce. To be honest, when I make a sauce I simply go to the refrigerator and use what I have. I sometimes discover that I design the sauce around the flavors I am craving. They all start off with… oil, vinegar, sugar (sugar substitute) and wine… then I am off to the races. Use your imagination to create your own sauce and write your own recipe.

Notes from Within: _____

_____
_____
_____
_____
_____
_____
_____
_____
_____
_____
_____
_____
_____
_____
_____

SUMMER MANGO SALSA

Notes from Within: _____

1 large ripe mango, diced
1 cup chopped fresh pineapple
1 vine ripe tomato, chopped
¼ cup diced scallions
¼ cup chopped fresh cilantro
2 teaspoons freshly squeezed lime juice

1. In a large mixing bowl, place mango, pineapple, tomato, scallions and cilantro. Cover with lime juice.

2. Refrigerate and keep for up to three days.

MINT CHUTNEY

4 Serrano green chilies, chopped
½ cup diced red onion
6 garlic cloves, crushed
½ cup chopped fresh cilantro leaves
2 cups chopped fresh mint leaves
2 teaspoons cumin seeds
3 teaspoons freshly squeezed lime juice

1. Combine chiles, onion, garlic, cilantro, mint, cumin seeds and lime juice in a blender and puree.

2. This chutney can be refrigerated for up to three days.

Notes from Within: _____

PINEAPPLE CAPER PEPPER SALSA

1 fresh ripe pineapple, chopped
2 vine ripe tomatoes, diced
½ cup diced apples
½ cup halved green grapes
1 small red onion, diced
½ cup diced cucumber
2 cups freshly squeezed lemon juice
½ cup capers
freshly ground black pepper to taste

1. Chop pineapple, tomatoes, apples, grapes, onion and cucumber. Place in mixing bowl, cover with lemon juice.
2. Toss in capers and add pepper to taste.

Notes from Within: _____

TAHINI SALAD DRESSING

¼ cup tahini
1 tablespoon honey
¼ cup olive oil
2 tablespoons freshly squeezed lemon juice

1 Combine tahini, honey, oil and lemon juice. Blend in a food processor or blender.

Notes from Within: _____

_____
_____
_____
_____
_____
_____
_____
_____
_____
_____
_____
_____
_____
_____
_____

PINEAPPLE SAUCE

2 cups fresh pineapple juice
1 cup soy sauce
¼ cup maple syrup
½ cup crushed fresh or frozen pineapple
2 cloves garlic, crushed
2 tablespoons strawberry jelly
1 tablespoon chopped fresh ginger
1 tablespoon sesame oil
½ teaspoon raw apple cider vinegar
black pepper to taste

1. In a saucepan, bring to a boil pineapple juice, soy sauce, maple syrup, pineapple, garlic, jelly, ginger, sesame oil, vinegar and pepper.
2. Cook for 20 minutes to reduce mixture.

Notes from Within: _____

GRAPE SAUCE

1 tablespoon ghee or butter
2 tablespoons chicken broth
¼ pound red grapes

1. In a saucepan, melt butter over medium heat and add broth.
2. Stir in grapes and simmer for 30 minutes.
3. Puree in blender.

> *Tip: This grape sauce really "wakes up" a piece of fish!*

Notes from Within: _____

SPICY CILANTRO SAUCE

Tip: Serve over halibut for a tasty dinner.

Notes from Within: _____

2 shallots, roasted
1 teaspoon olive oil
1 cup chopped fresh cilantro
1 cup chopped fresh parsley
3 garlic cloves, crushed
2 teaspoons grated fresh ginger root
½ teaspoon cumin seeds
½ teaspoon dried hot red pepper
2 tablespoons soy sauce
freshly squeezed lemon juice to taste

1. Brush shallots with olive oil, bake uncovered at 400°F for 10 minutes

2. Combine shallots, oil, cilantro, parsley, garlic, ginger, cumin seeds, red pepper, soy sauce and lemon juice in a food processor or blender. Puree until smooth.

3. Serve sauce warm.

GRAPEFRUIT SALSA

1 fresh cucumber, chopped
1 tablespoon chopped fresh dill weed
1 cup diced vine ripe tomatoes
1 tablespoon chopped scallions
1 cup chopped grapefruit
1 tablespoon freshly squeezed lemon juice
½ cup freshly squeezed orange juice

1. Combine cucumber, dill, tomatoes, scallions and grapefruit in large mixing bowl.
2. Cover with lemon and orange juice.
3. Keep in refrigerator for up to three days.

Notes from Within: _____

TANGERINE SAUCE

❄

Notes from Within: _____

6 tangerines, peeled, sectioned and halved
2 tablespoons maple syrup
1 cup freshly squeezed orange juice
1 tablespoon soy sauce
1 teaspoon cayenne pepper
1 tablespoon apple cider vinegar

1. Slice tangerine sections in half.

2. In a saucepan, combine tangerine pieces, maple syrup, orange juice, soy sauce, cayenne pepper and vinegar. Bring to a boil.

3. Reduce heat and simmer for 20 minutes to reduce mixture.

PEANUT SAUCE

6 cloves garlic, crushed

4 green onions, chopped

½ cup chopped fresh cilantro, remove stems

½ cup peanut butter

¼ cup tamari or soy sauce

2 tablespoons lemon juice

½ cup purified water

1 tablespoon freshly chopped ginger

1 In a blender or food processor, combine garlic, green onions, cilantro, peanut butter, tamari or soy sauce, lemon juice, water and ginger. Blend until smooth. If mixture becomes too thick, add water to thin.

Notes from Within: _____

HOMEMADE SMOKED CHIPOTLE CHILE BUTTER

Tip: Place this butter on anything and your taste buds will think they are in heaven. It is perfect for grilling.

1 cup ghee or butter
4–5 chipotle peppers, canned in adobo
6 cloves garlic, crushed
2 tablespoons chopped shallots
2 teaspoons freshly squeezed lime juice
sea salt and pepper to taste

1. Place ghee or butter, chipotle peppers, garlic, shallots, lime juice, sea salt and pepper in a food processor or blender and process until smooth. Scrape into a bowl and refrigerate for one hour.

2. Remove from refrigerator 20 minutes before using.

3. Use this butter on any seafood, meat or vegetable.

Notes from Within: _____

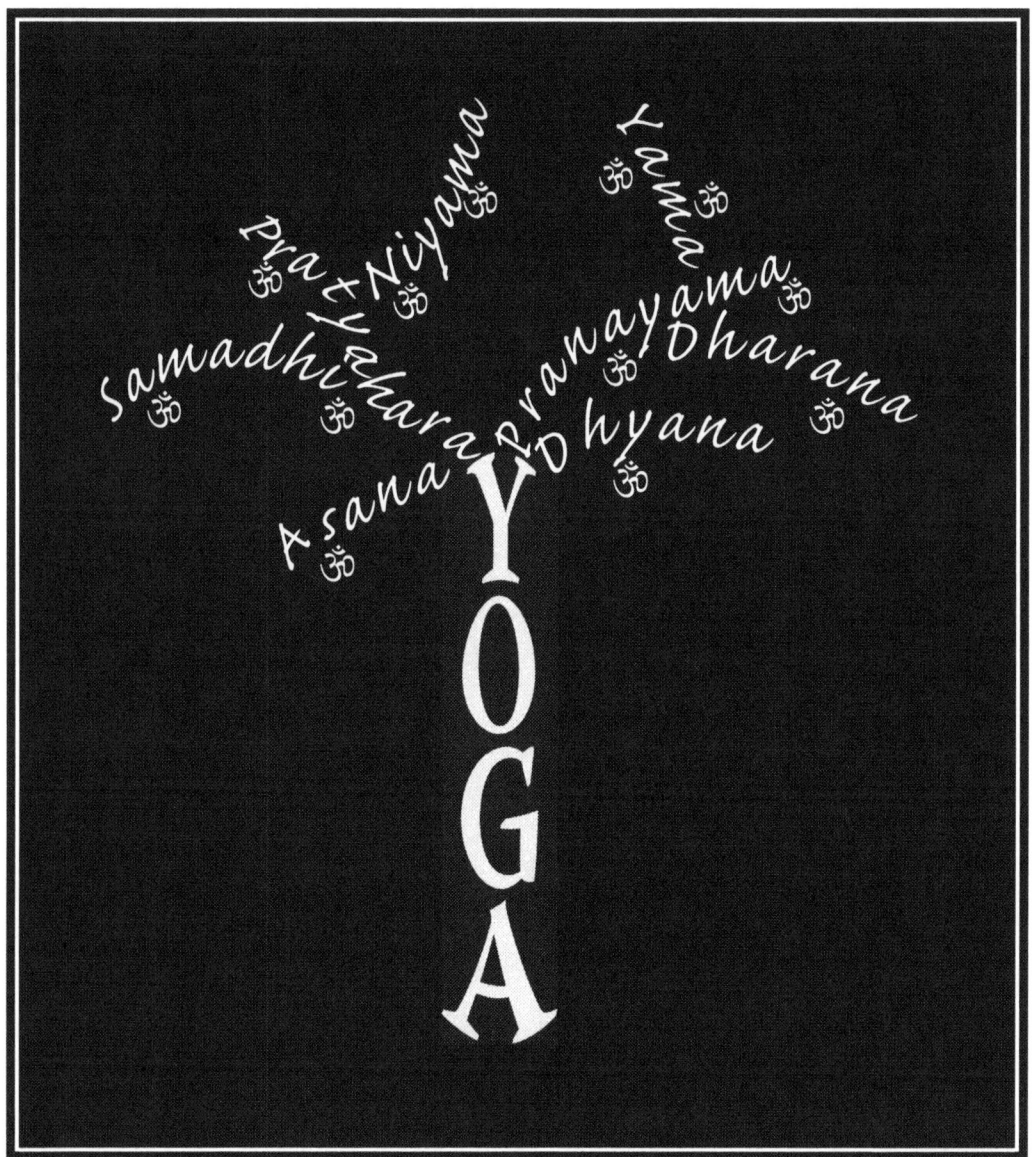

In my organic garden there sits a tree. This is a magical tree for me. This tree feeds me and keeps me on my spiritual path. My beautiful tree helps me from falling into too many of life's traps. My tree has eight violet limbs and many orange leaves. It is a wonder for all to see.

I love my little eight-limbed tree... by Jyl

Eight Limbs of Ashtanga Yoga

Yoga is a spiritual practice... "Don't you know that you are the temple of god... and that the Spirit of God dwells within you."

- *Apostle Paul*

The word Ashtanga means eight limbs (Ashtavangari). Think of the eight limbs like the ingredients of a recipe; each ingredient contributes to the whole character of the dish. I tell my Christian students, the eight limbs are like the Ten Commandments of the Bible. They are the spiritual guidelines or laws of life. Yogis from the ashtanga yoga practice believe the way to enlightenment is to understand, study and follow the eight limbs. The eight limbs are Yama, Niyama, Asana, Pranayama, Pratyahara, Dharana, Dhyana and Samadhi. Part of loving yourself to perfect health and loving your yoga practice is to celebrate these healthy steps, or eight limbs. The following briefly describes each of the eight limbs.

YAMA

Yama is the first limb, or path, that a yogi will set out to follow in his or her lifetime. This path represents non-violence, no lying, no stealing, no greed and no ego, as well as non-attachment to earthly goods, chastity (having sexual discernment) and moderation in all things. Do you know anyone who embodies this path? Use yoga to nourish a wider loving awareness that is present at all times. This limb teaches us to be impeccable with our thoughts, words and actions. We only have a lifetime to better ourselves, so it's time to cook up a new YOU!

NIYAMA

Niyama, or rules for living, addresses self-love. It is the attitude we have toward ourselves and includes our cleanliness, serenity, study, devotion and asceticism. Tapas is a part of this specific limb. Tapas means the food must be sattvic (pure), nirmala (untainted) and is never received with any form of unrighteousness. Also, the amount of food consumed should be observed by a yogi, and one should eat only as much food as is needed to sustain and maintain our bodies. The more yoga you do, the more you will come to understand this rule for living.

ASANA

Asana is doing the practice of yoga. Postures and breath help us to obtain greater awareness and awake us to our greater self. They also help to heal our bodies, releasing chronic muscular tension by freeing blocked energy. You start to become flexible and strong, not only in your body, but also in your mind and spirit. The asana practice is always done on an empty stomach. Remember to honor yourself after the practice with blessed food, cooked with love.

PRANAYAMA

Pranayama means expansion and an increase of the cosmic life-force energy. Practicing deep breathing works to energize and balance our mind-body connection. The minute you start to breathe, your mind clears, opening you to a spiritual source or spiritual experience. Stilling our minds allows us to connect with our true higher and greater existence. Allowing this spiritual experience to enter our minds is the first step in allowing it into our daily lives.

PRATYAHARA

Pratyahara is sometimes referred to as the withdrawal of senses. On the contrary, the more your senses have been refined, the greater the intensity of your senses. Think about food for example. The senses around smell, texture, color and taste can totally pass you by and go unnoticed. By going within to quiet the mind, you are creating greater space for observation of the senses. Dinner served after yoga allows a stilled mind and an open heart to perceive more and experience the joy of feeding your temple. Count on a heightened awareness when you are able to totally remove yourself from your everyday world. By unplugging yourself from the outside noise, you will have a greater sense of hearing.

DHARANA

Dharana is focusing the mind, or steadiness of the mind. Yoga creates a very strong physical core in our bodies, and the same is true about our minds. A strong clear mind will allow you to obtain more from daily life. An open mind will allow life to flow through you. You begin to see the gifts from the universe effortlessly coming to you. You will start to design the most beautiful meals from thoughts sent from above.

DHYANA

Dhyana is meditation. Meditation sets up greater communication between you and your God or higher power. Students meditate after we finish our asana practice. Sitting for 5 to 10 minutes is a great way to learn to meditate. Meditation is done twice a day, at sunrise and sunset. A clear mind will change your life. Every worry you have will become less of a worry. A mind that meditates is a clear and uncluttered mind.

SAMADHI

Samadhi is the most delicate state of awareness. It is how you feel when the cookies have just come hot out of the oven and there is a cold glass of milk waiting next to them. Samadhi is the ultimate state of self-realization and consciousness, when you know that if you eat the whole tray of cookies, you may not feel so good. This state leads to bliss, liberation and joy… so go ahead and eat the cookies!

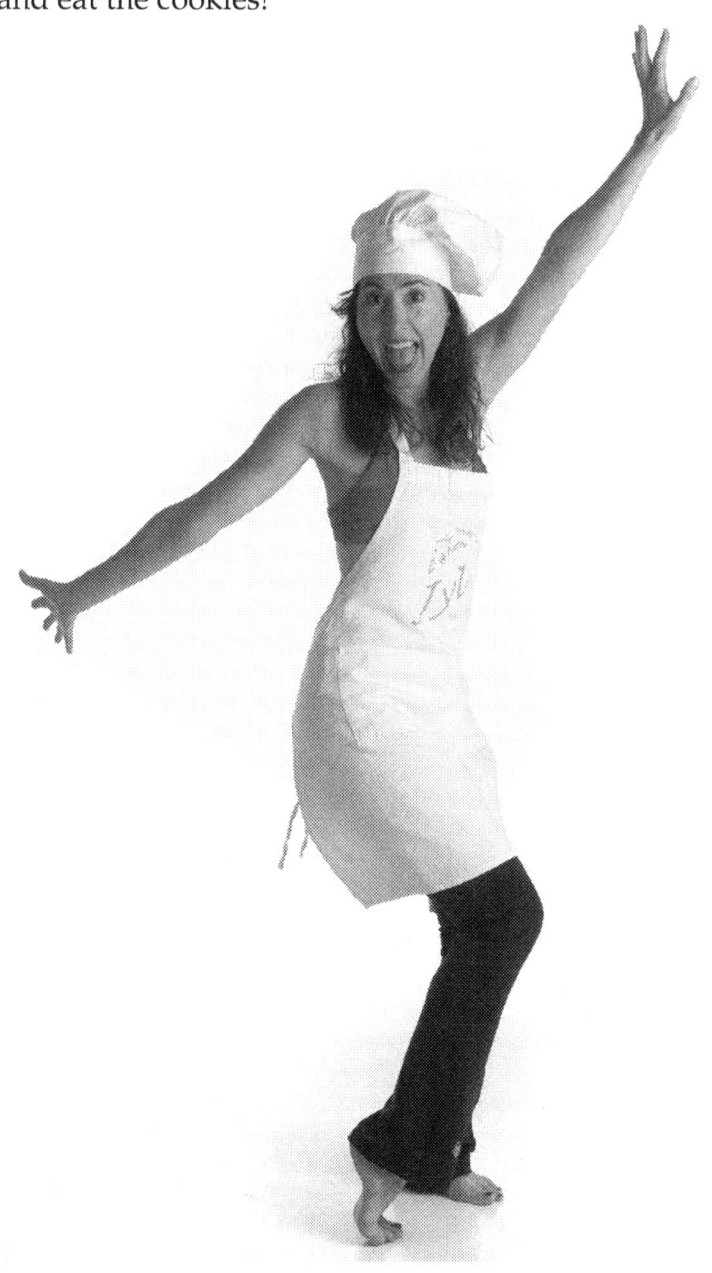

May the long time sun shine upon you

All love surround you

And the pure light within you

Guide your way on…

Sat Nam "truth is your identity"

Resources

RECOMMENDED READING

Ashtanga Yoga "The Practice Manual" by David Swenson

The Body Ecology Diet by Donna Gates
www.bodyecologydiet.com

Body, Mind, and Sport by John Douillard
www.randomhouse.com

Cleanse & Purify Thyself by Richard Anderson, N.D., N.M.D.

Cook Right for Your Type By Peter J. D'Adamo with Catherine Whitney

Delicious Living A Penton Publication
www.deliciouslivingmag.com

Living Yoga: Creating a Life Practice by Christy Turlington

Meditation As Medicine by Dharma Singh Khalsa, M.D. and Cameron Stauth

Reference Guide For Essential Oils by Connie and Alan Higley
abundanthealtheU@juno.com

The Secret of the Yamas A Spiritual Guide to Yoga by John McAfee

The Yeast Connection Cookbook by William Crook, M.D. & Marjorie Jones, R.N.

The Yoga Sutras Of Patanjali by Alistair Shearer

FOOD/OILS

Celtic Sea Salt available from the Grain & Salt Society, 800-867-7258
www.celtic-seasalt.com

Innerlight Supergreens distributed by Inner Light Inc., 801-655-0601
www.innerlightinc.com

Sambazon Acai berries, 877-726-2276
www.sambazon.com

Young Living Essential Oils available from Young Living, 800-371-3515
www.youngliving.com

WORKSHOPS

Workshops by Jyl Auxter: *What's Cooking Within, Cooking up a New You, Discover Your Dosha, Yoga and Women's Health, Balancing Your Chakras*
www.yogabyjyl.com

Flower Readings by Rick Jelusich
www.lightnews.org

Index

A

Acid foods 68-70
Acorn Squash with Millet 122
Alkaline foods 68-70
Almond, Cardamom and Nutmeg Brew, Warm 49
Arugula and Kale Salad 128
Aryans 13-14
Asana(s) 9, 13, 15, 19-20, 30, 202
Ashtanga 15, 201
Asian Noodle Salad with Toasted Sesame Dressing 127
Astringent foods 47, 48
Ayurvedic 41, 42

B

Balsamic Roasted Pears with Goat Cheese 168
Bandhas 15, 18
Basil Pesto 185
Beet(s),
    Cake with Cream Cheese Frosting 171
    Greens and Goat Cheese Ravioli 104
    Salad with Toasted Pumpkin Seeds 130
Bitter foods 48
Black Bean Soup 140
Blueberry Corn Muffins 160
Braised Baby Bok Choy 121
Bread,
    Blueberry Corn Muffins 160
    Goat-Cheese Popovers 159
    Pumpkin-Almond 161
Breakfast,
    French Toast 154
    Pancakes 153
    Kefir 156
    Love yourself Scrambled Eggs 155
Breath 15-16
Buddha 14, 16

C

C. Norman Shealy, M.D., Ph.D 16
Cake,
    Beet with Cream Cheese Frosting 171
    Chocolate Pudding 173
    Gingerbread 172
    Jyl's Famous Tofu Birthday 62, 178
    Strawberry Oatmeal 170
    Chocolate Tort 177
    Chocolate Truffle Tart 175
    White Chocolate Cheesecake 174
Carob Almond Cookies 166

Carrot(s),
    Asparagus and Tarragon 117
    Ginger Soup 149
    Watermelon Mashed 118
Celery Root Soup 141
Chakra(s) 11, 29-39
    Chakra 1 Muladhara 31
    Chakra 2 Svadhisthana 32
    Chakra 3 Manipuri 33
    Chakra 4 Anahata 34
    Chakra 5 Visuddhu 35
    Chakra 6 Ajna 36
    Chakra 7 Sahasrara 37
Chicken,
    Free Range and Buckwheat Soba Dish 108
    Grilled Skewers 110
    Healing Lemon Garlic Soup 137
    Love Rose Sauce with Chicken Breast 58
    Mustard with Thyme 106
    Thai with Peanuts 107
Chestnuts Roasting on an Open Fire Soup 146
Chocolate
    Crepes with Strawberry filling 169
    Ganache Sauce 62, 176
    Pudding Cake 173
    Tort 177
    Truffle Tart 175
Cooking 57
Courage 5, 6, 7, 17
Crab Cakes, Healing 92
Cucumber Kefir/Yogurt Soup 142

D

D'Adamo, Dr. Peter J. 67
Desserts,
    Balsamic Roasted Pears with Goat Cheese 168
    Carob Almond Cookies 166
    Chocolate Crepes with Strawberry filling 169
    Green Tea Poached Pears 167
    Lemon-Lime Tofu Creme Pie 165
    Pomegranate Soy Ice Cream 179
Dharana 202
Dhyana 203
Donna Gates 67
Dosha(s) 11, 41-53, 55, 85
    score 46
    test 43-45
    time 50-51
    workout 50
Dosha Pasta Dish 102-103

INDEX

D

Dr. Richard Jelusich 38
Drinks,
    Live Longer Smoothie by Jyl 72
    Purification Potion 48
    Rose Milkshake 49
    Sassy Saffron Cocktail 49
    Turmeric Tonic 48
    Warm Almond, Cardamom and Nutmeg Brew 49
    Yoga by Jyl Juice 71
Drishti 15, 19, 23

E

Eating to Heal 67
Edge(s) 15-17, 23
Essential oil(s) 51-54
    benefits of 53
    some common oils and their uses 53-54
Exercise 50

F

5 Minute Soup 147
Faith 6, 10, 11, 12
Flower readings 38
Foods, 47
    astringent 47, 48
    bitter 48
    pungent 48
    salty 47
    sour 47
    sweet foods 47
Freeman, Richard 19
Free Range Chicken and Buckwheat Soba Dish 108
French Toast 154

G

Garlic Mayonnaise 91
Gates, Donna 67
Ghee 67
Gingerbread Cake 172
Goat-Cheese Popovers 159
Go Within 77
Grapefruit Salsa 194
Grape Sauce 192
Green Tea Poached Pears 167
Grilled Chicken Skewers 110
Grilled Vegetables 115
Guru 14

H

Happiness 20, 75
Healing Crab Cakes 92
Healing Lemon Garlic Chicken Soup 137
Healthy Raw Salad 129
Hindus 18
Homemade Smoked Chipotle Chile Butter 197
How to create your own Yoga and Dinner Party 59

I

Iyanla Vanzant 2

J

Jelusich, Dr. Richard 38
Jesus 16
Juicing 71
Jyl's Famous Tofu Birthday Cake 62, 178

K

Kapha(s) 42, 45, 47-50, 85
Kefir 68, 156

L

Lemon-Lime Tofu Creme Pie 165
Linguine with Chard and Pine Nuts 105
Live Longer Smoothie by Jyl 72
Love Rose Sauce with Chicken Breast 58
Love yourself Scrambled Eggs 155
Lycopenes 71

M

Meditation, 11, 25, 26-27, 50, 51, 75
    benefits of 26
Millet,
    Acorn Squash with 122
    Cakes 123
Mint,
    Garlic Salad Dressing 183
    Chutney 188
Muffins,
    Blueberry Corn 160
    Goat-Cheese Popovers 159
Mustard,
    Basil Salad Dressing 184
    Chicken with Thyme 106

N

Niyama 202
New Life Cleanse, A 76

INDEX

O

Ocean Foods 84

P

Pan-fried Scallops with Truffle and Grape Sauce 99
Pancakes 153
Pasta,
    Asian Noodle Salad 127
    Beet Greens and Goat Cheese Ravioli 104
    Dosha Pasta Dish 102-103
    Free Range Chicken and Buckwheat Soba Dish 108
    Linguine with Chard and Pine Nuts 105
Patanjali 13
Peanut Sauce 109, 196
Pea,
    Bisque with Fresh Tarragon and Shrimp 136
    Pancakes 124
Phoenix Rising 21
Pineapple,
    Caper Pepper Salsa 189
    Sauce 191
Pistachio-Salmon 98
Pitta(s) 42, 44, 46, 47, 48, 49, 50, 85
Pomegranate Soy Ice Cream 179
Portabella & Shiitake Mushrooms on Arugula Salad 131
Potlatch Stew 139
Prana 15, 18
Pranayama 202
Pratyahara 202
Prayer Beans 120
Presentation 62, 83, 84
Pumpkin,
    Almond Bread 161
    Vegetable Tofu Stir-fry 119
    Soup 135
Pungent foods 47-48
Purification Potion 48

Q

Quan Yin 42

R

Raindrop Therapy 21
Raspberry Chipotle Sauce 93
Red Curry Lentil Soup 144
Reiki 21, 57
Resnick, Stella, Ph.D. 20
Rice, Saffron 114
Richard Freeman 19
Rose Milkshake 49

S

Saffron Rice 114
Salad,
    Arugula and Kale 128
    Asian Noodle with Toasted Sesame Dressing 127
    Beet with Toasted Pumpkin Seeds 130
    Healthy Raw 129
    Portabella & Shiitake Mushrooms on Arugula 131
    Mint Garlic Dressing 183
    Mustart Basil Dressing 184
    Tahini Dressing 190
Salmon,
    Cakes 90
    Pistachio 98
    Smoked and Cream Cheese Soup 148
    Stack 94-97
    Thai Coconut Curried with Greens 61, 89
Salty foods 47
Samadhi 203
Sambazon Acai 72
Sassy Saffron Cocktail 49
Sauce,
    Basil Pesto 185
    Carob Mole with Almonds & Sesame Seeds 113
    Chocolate Ganache 62, 176
    Garlic Mayonnaise 91
    Grapefruit Salsa 194
    Grape 192
    Homemade Smoked Chipotle Chile Butter 197
    Mint Chutney 188
    Peanut 109, 196
    Pineapple Caper Pepper Salsa 189
    Pineapple 191
    Raspberry Chipotle 93
    Saucy Sauces for Sassy Students 186
    Spicy Cilantro 193
    Summer Mango Salsa 111, 187
    Tangerine 195
Self love test 77
Shealy, C. Norman, M.D., Ph.D 16
Shellfish,
    Healing Crab Cakes 92
    Pan-fried Scallops with Truffle and Grape Sauce 99
    Potlatch Stew 139
    Risotto 101
    Shrimp and Scallop Kabobs 100
Smoked Salmon and Cream Cheese Soup 148
Some common oils and their uses 53-54

INDEX

S

Soup,
   5 Minute 147
   Black Bean 140
   Carrot Ginger 149
   Celery Root 141
   Chestnuts Roasting on an Open Fire 146
   Cucumber Kefir/Yogurt 142
   Healing Lemon Garlic Chicken 137
   Pea Bisque with Fresh Tarragon and Shrimp 136
   Potlatch Stew 139
   Pumpkin 135
   Red Curry Lentil 144
   Smoked Salmon and Cream Cheese 148
   Sweet Potato and Rosemary 143
   Vegetable 138
   Wild Mushroom 145
Sour foods 47
Spicy Cilantro Sauce 193
Spinach and Asparagus 116
Sprouts 70
Starting Over 6
Stella Resnick, Ph.D. 20
Stevia 68
Strawberry Oatmeal Cake 170
Summer Mango Salsa 111, 187
Supplements 84
Sweet foods 47
Sweet Potato and Rosemary Soup 143

T

Tahini Salad Dressing 190
Tangerine Sauce 195
Thai,
   Chicken with Peanuts 107
   Coconut Curried Salmon with Greens 61, 89
Theta Healing 21
Trans fat(s) 65-67
Tri-dosha(s) 42, 46
Turkey,
   Carob Mole with Almonds & Sesame Seeds 112-113
Turmeric Tonic 48

U

Ujjayi breathing 15, 18

V

Vanzant, Iyanla 2
Vatta(s) 42, 43, 46, 47, 50, 51, 85
Vegetable(s),
   Acorn Squash with Millet 122
   Braised Baby Bok Choy 121
   Carrots, Asparagus and Tarragon 117
   Grilled 115
   Pea Pancakes 124
   Prayer Beans 120
   Pumpkin Vegetable Tofu Stir-fry 119
   Soup 138
   Spinach and Asparagus 116
   Watermelon Mashed Carrots 118

W

Warm Almond, Cardamom and Nutmeg Brew 49
Watermelon juice 71
Watermelon Mashed Carrots 118
White Chocolate Cheesecake 174
Wild Mushroom Soup 145

Y

Yama 201
Yoga, 7, 10, 11, 13-22, 25, 30, 50, 66, 75
   basic components of 15
   benefits of 15
   and dinner 57, 58, 59, 60, 63, 83
   How to create your own Yoga and Dinner Party 59
   history 13
   perfect workout, the 14
   picking a perfect teacher 10
   therapy 15, 20-21
   teacher(s) 1, 7, 9, 10, 14, 17, 20, 59
Yoga by Jyl Juice 71

www.ingramcontent.com/pod-product-compliance
Lightning Source LLC
Chambersburg PA
CBHW081938170426
43202CB00018B/2940